The Vibrant Keto Diet Desserts for Beginners

Quick, Easy and Delicious Keto Diet Dessert Recipes to Burn Fat and Enjoy your Diet

Jessica Simpson

© **Copyright 2020 - All rights reserved.**

The content contained within this book may not be reproduced, duplicated or transmitted without direct written permission from the author or the publisher.

Under no circumstances will any blame or legal responsibility be held against the publisher, or author, for any damages, reparation, or monetary loss due to the information contained within this book. Either directly or indirectly.

Legal Notice:

This book is copyright protected. This book is only for personal use. You cannot amend, distribute, sell, use, quote or paraphrase any part, or the content within this book, without the consent of the author or publisher.

Disclaimer Notice:

Please note the information contained within this document is for educational and entertainment purposes only. All effort has been executed to present accurate, up to date, and reliable, complete information. No warranties of any kind are declared or implied. Readers acknowledge that the author is not engaging in the rendering of legal, financial, medical or professional advice. The content within this book has been derived from various sources. Please consult a licensed professional before attempting any techniques outlined in this book.

By reading this document, the reader agrees that under no circumstances is the author responsible for any losses, direct or indirect, which are incurred as a result of the use of information contained within this document, including, but not limited to, — errors, omissions, or inaccuracies.

Contents

Raspberry Tart 11

Blackberry Lemon Tart 13

Peanut Butter Pie 15

Mixed Berries Tart 18

Blueberry Lemon Filling Tart 20

Berries And Mascarpone Cream Tart 23

Easy Strawberry Pie 25

Pumpkin Almond Pie 27

Lemon Curd Tart With Blackberries 30

Delicious Blueberry Pie 32

Low-carb Keto Tarts With Berries And Mascarpone Cream 34

Strawberry Cream Pie 37

Delicious Custard Tarts 39

Butter Pie 41

Crust-less Pumpkin Pie 44

Almond Meal Vanilla Tart 46

Keto Lemon Curd Tarts With Blackberries 48

Apple Tart 51

Strawberry Vanilla Tart 53

Cheesecake Tarts 55

Dark Chocolate Tart 57

Blueberry Lemon 60

Lemon Meringue Pie 63

Grasshopper Pie 66

Lemon Pie 68

Quick & Simple Strawberry Tart 70

Easy Lemon Pie 72

Chocolate Keto Pudding 74

Fruit And Cheese 76

Low Carb Lemon Tart 78

Cheesecake Jam Tarts 80

Mock Apple Pie 82

Strawberry Pie With Gelatin 84

Pumpkin Pie 86

Strawberry Tart 88

Cookie Pie 91

Low Carb Vanilla Pudding 93

Strawberry Mascarpone Tart 96

Key Lime Pie 98

Mascarpone Tart 100

Delicious Pumpkin Cream Pie 103

Flavorful Strawberry Cream Pie 105

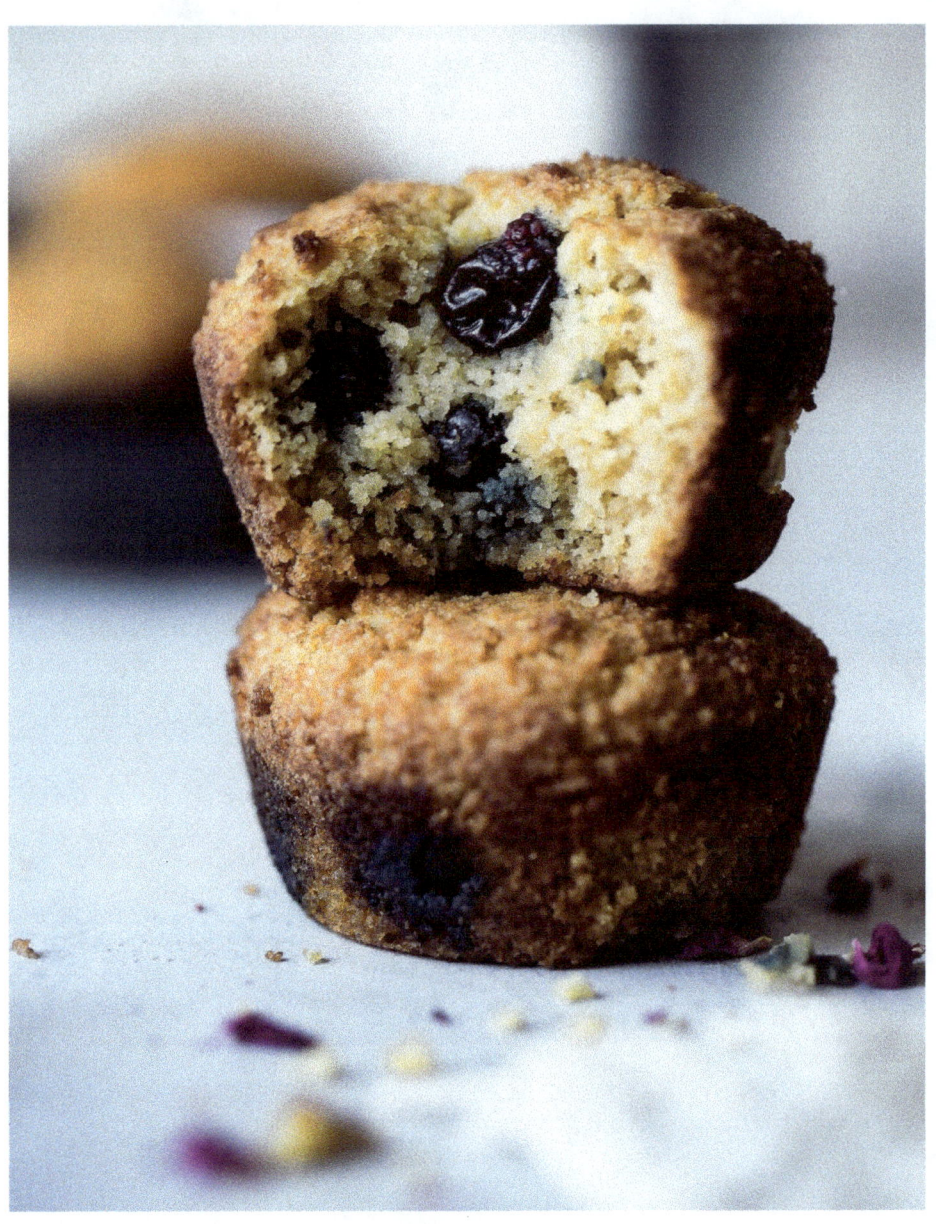

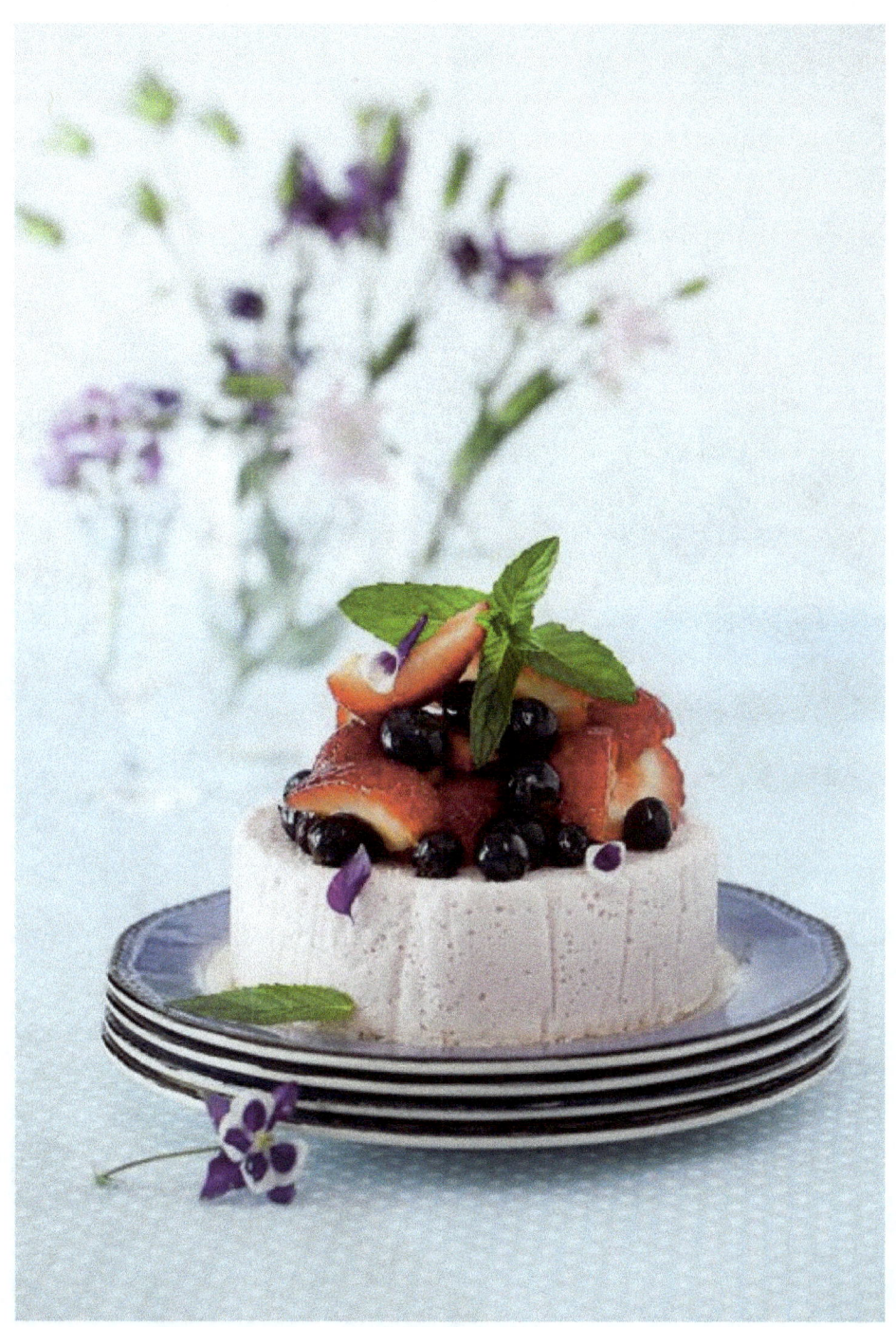

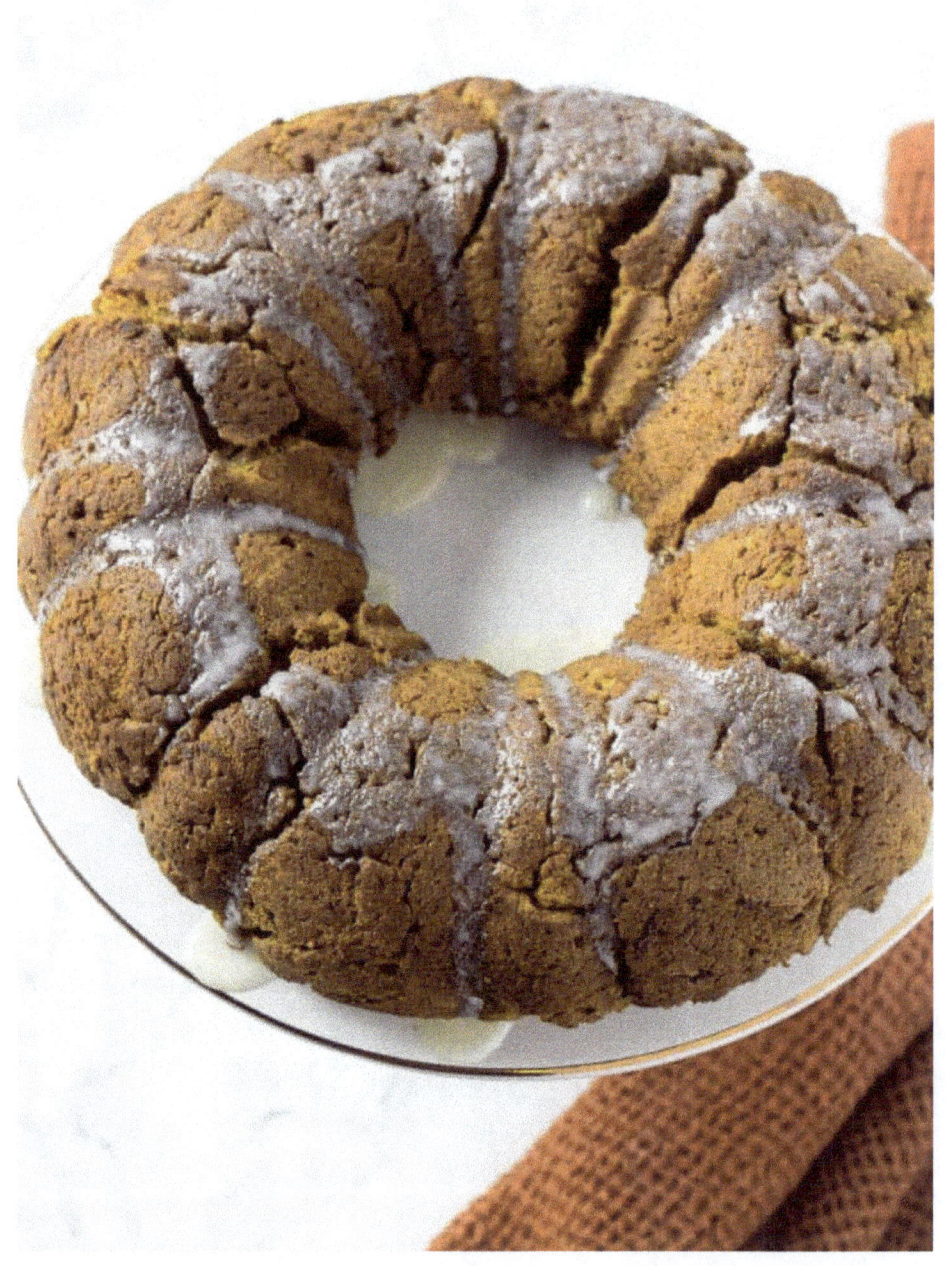

Raspberry Tart

Servings: 4

Cooking Time: 23 Minutes

Ingredients:

- 5 egg whites
- 2 cups raspberries
- ½ cup butter, melted
- 1 tsp baking powder
- 1 tsp vanilla
- 1 lemon zest, grated
- 1 cup almond flour
- ½ cup xylitol

Directions:

1. Preheat the oven to 375 F 0 C.
2. Grease tart tin with cooking spray and set aside.
3. In a large bowl, whisk egg whites until foamy.
4. Add sweetener, baking powder, vanilla, lemon zest, and almond flour and mix until well combined.
5. Add melted butter and stir well.
6. Pour batter in prepared tart tin and top with raspberries.
7. Bake in preheated oven for 20-23 minutes.
8. Serve and enjoy.

Nutrition Info: Per Servings: Net Carbs: 4.2g; Calories: 213 Total Fat: 18.8g; Saturated Fat: 7.8g Protein: 5.8g; Carbs: 7.; Fiber: 3.7g; Sugar: 2.3g; Fat 81% Protein 11% Carbs 8%

Blackberry Lemon Tart

Servings: 8

Cooking Time: 15 Minutes

Ingredients:
- 1 cup lemon curd
- 1 cup blackberries
- 1 tablespoon sliced almonds
- 2 9" tart molds with loose bottoms
- Almond Flour Pie Crust
- 1.5 cup blanched almond flour
- 1/2 cup coconut flour
- 4 tablespoons erythritol, powdered
- 2 eggs
- 4 tablespoons cold butter, unsalted

Directions:
1. Let your oven preheat at 350 degrees F.
2. Prepare the dough by mixing everything for pie crust.
3. Divide the dough into two equal sized balls.
4. Take two tart molds and layer it with foil and parchment paper.
5. Spread one dough ball into each pan and press it evenly.
6. Make a few holes into each dough layer using a fork.
7. Bake the tart crusts for 15 mins in the preheated oven.

8. Place the tart pans on a wire pan to cool the crust at room temperature.
9. Fill both the crusts with lemon curd equally.
10. Top it with berries, erythritol and almond slices.
11. Serve and enjoy.

Nutrition Info: Calories 321 ;Total Fat 9 g ;Saturated Fat 5.1 g ;Cholesterol 17 mg ;Sodium 28 mg ;Total Carbs 8.1 g ;Sugar 1.8 g ;Fiber 0.4 g ;Protein 5.4 g

Peanut Butter Pie

Servings: 16

Cooking Time: 10 Minutes

Ingredients:
- For crust:
- ¾ cup almond flour
- ½ cup of cocoa powder
- ½ cup erythritol
- 13 cup almond butter
- ½ cup butter softened
- For filling:
- 1 ½ cups heavy whipping cream
- ½ cup erythritol
- 13 cup peanut butter
- 8 oz cream cheese, softened

Directions:
1. For the crust: In a large bowl, combine together butter, cocoa powder, sweetener, and almond butter until smooth.
2. Add almond flour and beat until mixture stiff.
3. Transfer crust mixture into the greased spring-form cake pan and spread evenly and place in the refrigerator for 15- minutes.

4. Meanwhile for filling: In a mixing bowl, beat sweetener, peanut butter, and cream cheese until smooth.
5. Add heavy cream and beat until stiff peaks form.
6. Spread filling mixture in prepared crust and refrigerate for 2 hours.
7. Slice and serve.

Nutrition Info: Per Servings: Net Carbs: 2.7g; Calories: 209; Total Fat: 20.7g; Saturated Fat: 10.3g Protein: 4.4g; Carbs: 4.4g; Fiber: 1.7g; Sugar: 0.; Fat 88% Protein 7% Carbs 5%

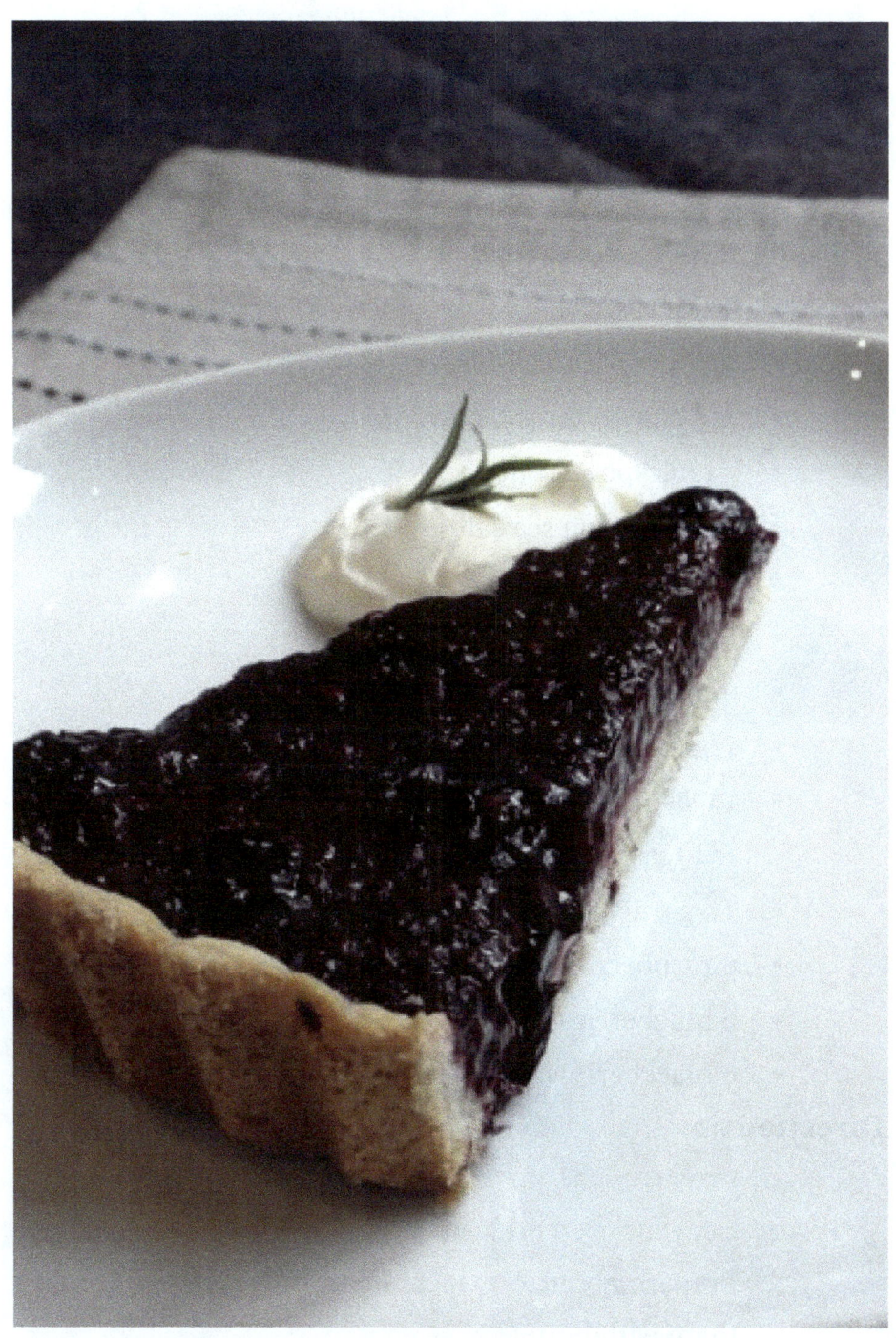

Mixed Berries Tart

Servings: 8

Cooking Time: 10 Minutes

Ingredients:

- Tart crust:
- 2 1/4 cups almond flour
- 1/4 cup erythritol, powdered
- 5 tablespoons butter, melted
- 1/4 teaspoon sea salt
- Filling
- 6 oz. mascarpone cheese
- 2 tablespoons erythritol
- 1/3 cup heavy cream
- 1 teaspoon vanilla essence
- 1/4 teaspoon lemon zest fresh
- To garnish:
- 6 raspberries
- 6 blueberries
- 6 blackberries

Directions:

1. Crust:
2. Let your oven preheat at 350 degrees F.
3. Prepare about 6 4 inch small tart pans by greasing them with butter.

4. Combine butter with almond flour, sweetener, and salt in a food processor.
5. Divide this coarse mixture into the prepared pan and press them firmly.
6. Use the fork to make a few holes in each pan.
7. Bake the tart crust for 10 minutes until golden around edges.
8. Filling:
9. Beat the cream with erythritol in an electric mixer for 2 minutes approximately.
10. Gradually stir in cream and continue beating until the mixture thickens.
11. Stir in lemon zest and vanilla essence.
12. Spread this filling in the baked crust of each tart pan.
13. Garnish with berries and chill for 10 minutes in the refrigerator.
14. Serve and enjoy.

Nutrition Info: Calories 237 ;Total Fat 22 g ;Saturated Fat 9 g ;Cholesterol 35 mg ;Sodium 118 mg ;Total Carbs 5 g ;Sugar 1 g ;Fiber 2 g ;Protein 5 g

Blueberry Lemon Filling Tart

Servings: 8

Cooking Time: 25 Minutes

Ingredients:
- Crust:
- 1 cup superfine almond flour
- 2 tablespoons swerve
- 3/4 teaspoon baking powder
- 1 pinch sea salt
- 1 teaspoon vanilla essence
- 4 tablespoons extra cold butter
- Filling:
- 8-ounce cream cheese
- 3 tablespoons erythritol
- 1 large egg
- 1/2 teaspoon lemon essence
- 1 teaspoon lemon zest fresh
- Topping:
- 1 cup blueberries fresh or frozen

Directions:
1. Blend butter with salt, almond flour, and erythritol in a suitable bowl.
2. Spread this mixture in an 8inch pan layered with wax paper.

3. Bake the tart crust for 20 minutes in a preheated oven at 0 degrees.
4. Place the crust pan on wire rack for 10 minutes to cool at room temperature.
5. Whisk lemon juice, lemon zest, ¾ cup almond flour, salt, and ¾ cup erythritol.
6. Once combined, pour this mixture into the baked crust and spread it evenly.
7. Return the pan to the oven again for 25 minutes at the same temperature.
8. Garnish with blueberries.
9. Serve and enjoy.

Nutrition Info: Calories 367 ;Total Fat 35.1 g ;Saturated Fat 1 g ;Cholesterol 12 mg ;Sodium 48 mg ;Total Carbs 8.9 g ;Sugar 3.8 g ;Fiber 2.1 g ;Protein 6.3 g

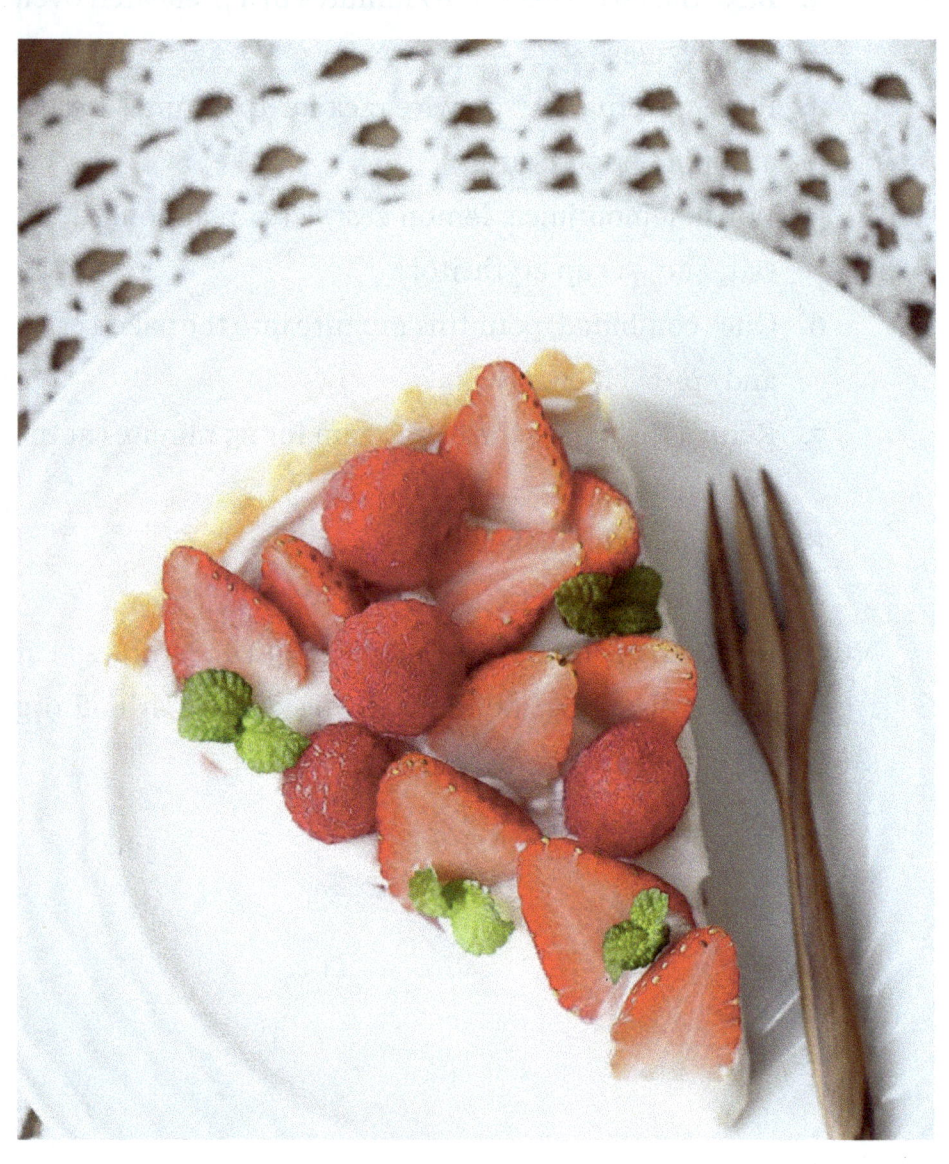

Berries And Mascarpone Cream Tart

Servings: 6

Cooking Time: 30 Minutes

Ingredients:

- For the Tart Crust:
- 2 1/4 cups almond flour
- 1/4 teaspoon sea salt
- 1/4 cup erythritol sweetener
- 5 tablespoons melted butter
- For the Mascarpone Cream:
- 2 tablespoons erythritol sweetener
- 1/4 teaspoon lemon zest
- 1 teaspoon vanilla extract, unsweetened
- 6-ounce mascarpone cheese, full-fat
- 1/3 cup heavy cream
- For Garnishing:
- 6 raspberries
- 3 strawberries, halved
- 6 blueberries
- 6 blackberries

Directions:

1. Set oven to 350 degrees F and let preheat.
2. In the meantime, grease six tart pan, each about 4-inch, and set aside.

3. Prepare the crust and for this, stir together all the ingredients for crust until incorporated.
4. Divide evenly between the prepared tart pan and press down evenly, down the walls and bottom.
5. Use a fork to make holes in the dough and then place pan into the oven to bake for 8 to 10 minutes or until nicely golden brown.
6. When done, place tart pans on wire rack and cool completely.
7. Meanwhile, prepare mascarpone cream and for this, place cheese in a bowl, then add sweetener and beat with an electric mixer for 2 minutes at low speed. Slowly beat in cream, then increase mixer speed to medium and continue beating for 30 to 60 seconds or until thick.
8. Then beat in lemon zest and vanilla until mixed.
9. Spoon the filling into prepared tarts, smooth with top and top with berries.
10. Serve straightaway.

Nutrition Info: Calories: 237 Cal, Carbs: 5 g, Fat: 22 g, Protein: 5 g, Fiber: 2 g.

Easy Strawberry Pie

Servings: 8

Cooking Time: 10 Minutes

Ingredients:
- For crust:
- 2 tbsp butter, melted
- 1 cup pecans, chopped
- 1 tsp liquid stevia
- For filling:
- ½ tsp vanilla
- 23 cup Swerve
- 1 cup strawberries, chopped
- 1 ½ cup heavy whipping cream
- 8 oz cream cheese, softened

Directions:
1. Preheat the oven to 350 F 0 C.
2. Add pecans in food processor and process until if finely crush.
3. Add sweetener and butter in crushed pecans and process until well combined.
4. Greased pie pan with butter.
5. Add crust mixture into the greased pie pan and spread evenly. Using back of spoon smooth the pecan mixture.

6. Bake in preheated oven for 10 minutes.
7. Allow to cool completely.
8. For the filling: In a large bowl, beat heavy whipping cream until stiff peaks form.
9. In another bowl, add strawberries, vanilla, sweetener, and cream cheese and beat until smooth.
10. Add heavy cream in strawberry mixture and beat until smooth.
11. Pour strawberry cream mixture into crust and spread well.
12. Place in refrigerator for 2 hours.
13. Slice and serve.

Nutrition Info: Per Servings: Net Carbs: 3.1g; Calories: 3 Total Fat: 32.2g; Saturated Fat: 14.2g Protein: 4.3g; Carbs: 5g; Fiber: 1.9g; Sugar: 1.5g; Fat 92% Protein 5% Carbs 3%

Pumpkin Almond Pie

Servings: 8

Cooking Time: 57 Minutes

Ingredients:
- Almond Flour Pie Crust
- 2 cups almond flour
- 4 tablespoons butter, melted
- 1 teaspoon vanilla
- 1 egg yolk
- ½ teaspoon cinnamon
- Pumpkin Spice Filling
- 8 ounces cream cheese
- 1 cup heavy cream
- 4 eggs
- 1 teaspoon vanilla
- 2 teaspoons pumpkin pie spice
- ¼ teaspoon salt
- ⅔ cups Swerve (Confectioners)

Directions:
1. Put everything for the crust in a suitable bowl.
2. Spread and press this mixture into a pie pan.
3. Bake this crust for 12 minutes in a preheated oven at 400 degrees F.
4. Filling

5. Beat eggs in the cream cheese until it turns frothy.
6. Add rest of the ingredients to the cream cheese and stir well to combine.
7. Spread this filling into the baked crust evenly.
8. Return the stuffed pie to the oven and bake for another 45 minutes at the same temperature.
9. Place the hot pie on a wire rack to cool for 10 minutes.
10. Garnish with almond or as desired.
11. Slice and enjoy.

Nutrition Info: Calories 285 ;Total Fat 27.3 g ;Saturated Fat 14.5 g ;Cholesterol 175 mg ;Sodium 165 mg ;Total Carbs 3.5 g ;Sugar 0.4 g ;Fiber 0.9 g ;Protein 7.2 g

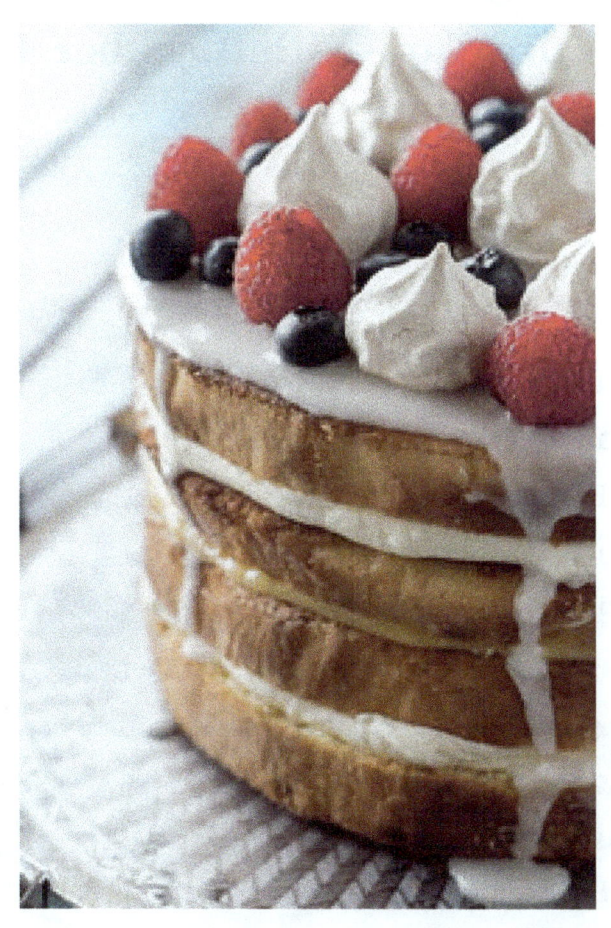

Lemon Curd Tart With Blackberries

Servings: 12

Cooking Time: 35 Minutes

Ingredients:

- 12-ounce blackberries
- 1 tablespoon sliced almonds
- 1 cup lemon curd, chilled
- For Pie Crust:
- 1 ½ cup almond flour
- ½ cup coconut flour
- 4 tablespoons erythritol sweetener
- 4 tablespoons unsalted butter, chilled
- 2 eggs

Directions:

1. Set oven to 350 degrees F and let preheat.
2. In the meantime, prepare the crust and for this, place all the ingredients for crust in a large bowl, stir well and knead for 3 minutes or more until dough comes together.
3. Take two 9-inch tart pan and grease with oil and line with a parchment sheet.
4. Divide dough into two portions, add each portion to the tart pan and spread evenly throughout the pan.

5. Place pan into the oven and bake for 1minutes or until crusts are nicely browned.
6. Let baked crusts cool completely, then add lemon curd in it and cover with berries and lemon slices.
7. Serve straightaway.

Nutrition Info: Calories: 216 Cal, Carbs: 10.6 g, Fat: 19.9 g, Protein: 7.7 g, Fiber: 5.7 g.

Delicious Blueberry Pie

Servings: 8

Cooking Time: 25 Minutes

Ingredients:

- For crust:
- 4 eggs
- 1 tbsp water
- ¼ tsp baking powder
- 1 ½ cups coconut flour
- 1 cup butter, melted
- Pinch of salt
- For filling:
- 8 oz cream cheese
- 2 tbsp swerve
- 1 ½ cup fresh blueberries

Directions:

1. Spray 9-inch pie pan with cooking spray and set aside.
2. In a large bowl, mix together all crust ingredients until dough is formed.
3. Divide dough in half and roll out I between two parchment paper sheet and set aside.
4. Preheat the oven to 350 F 180 C.
5. Transfer one crust sheet into greased pie pan.
6. Spread cream cheese on crust.

7. Mix together blueberries and sweetener. Spread blueberries on top of the cream cheese layer.
8. Cover pie with other half rolled crust and bake for 25 minutes.
9. Allow to cool completely then slice and serve.

Nutrition Info: Per Servings: Net Carbs: 5.4g; Calories: 362 Total Fat: 35.6g; Saturated Fat: 21.9g Protein: 5.7g; Carbs: 7g; Fiber: 1.6g; Sugar: 3.1g; Fat 88% Protein 6% Carbs 6%

Low-carb Keto Tarts With Berries And Mascarpone Cream

Servings: 6

Cooking Time: 15 Minutes

Ingredients:
- For crust:
- 1 cup + 2 tablespoons almond flour
- 2 ½ tablespoons salted butter, melted
- 2 tablespoons powdered erythritol
- For mascarpone cream:
- 3 ounces mascarpone, at room temperature
- ½ teaspoon vanilla extract
- 1 tablespoon powdered Swerve or erythritol
- 3 tablespoons heavy cream
- 1/8 teaspoon grated, fresh lemon zest
- For topping:
- 2 strawberries, chopped
- A handful mixed berries (blueberries, raspberries and blackberries)

Directions:
1. Add all the ingredients for crust into a bowl and mix well.
2. Grease 6 mini tart pans with oil. Divide the dough into 6 equal portions and place in the pans. Press the dough

well onto the bottom as well as sides of the pans. Place the pans in the freezer for about 5-8 minutes.
3. Remove pans from the freezer and prick the crusts with a fork in a few places.
4. Bake in a preheated oven 350° F for about 8 – 10 minutes or until light brown.
5. Remove from the oven and let cool.
6. Meanwhile, make the mascarpone cream as follows: Add mascarpone and sweetener into a mixing bowl. Set the electric hand mixer on low speed and beat the mixture for 2 minutes.
7. Add cream and continue beating on the same speed for about a minute.
8. Beat on medium speed for 30 – 60 seconds. It will thicken. Do not over beat, otherwise the cream will separate into curd-like, tiny pieces. Be very careful during the last couple of minutes of beating.
9. Add lemon zest and vanilla and fold gently.
10. Transfer the mascarpone cream into a piping bag. Pipe it over the mini tarts.
11. Divide the berries among the tarts and serve.

Nutrition Info: Per Servings: Calories: 222 kcal, Fat: 20.2 g, Carbohydrates: 5.8 g, Protein: 5.2 g

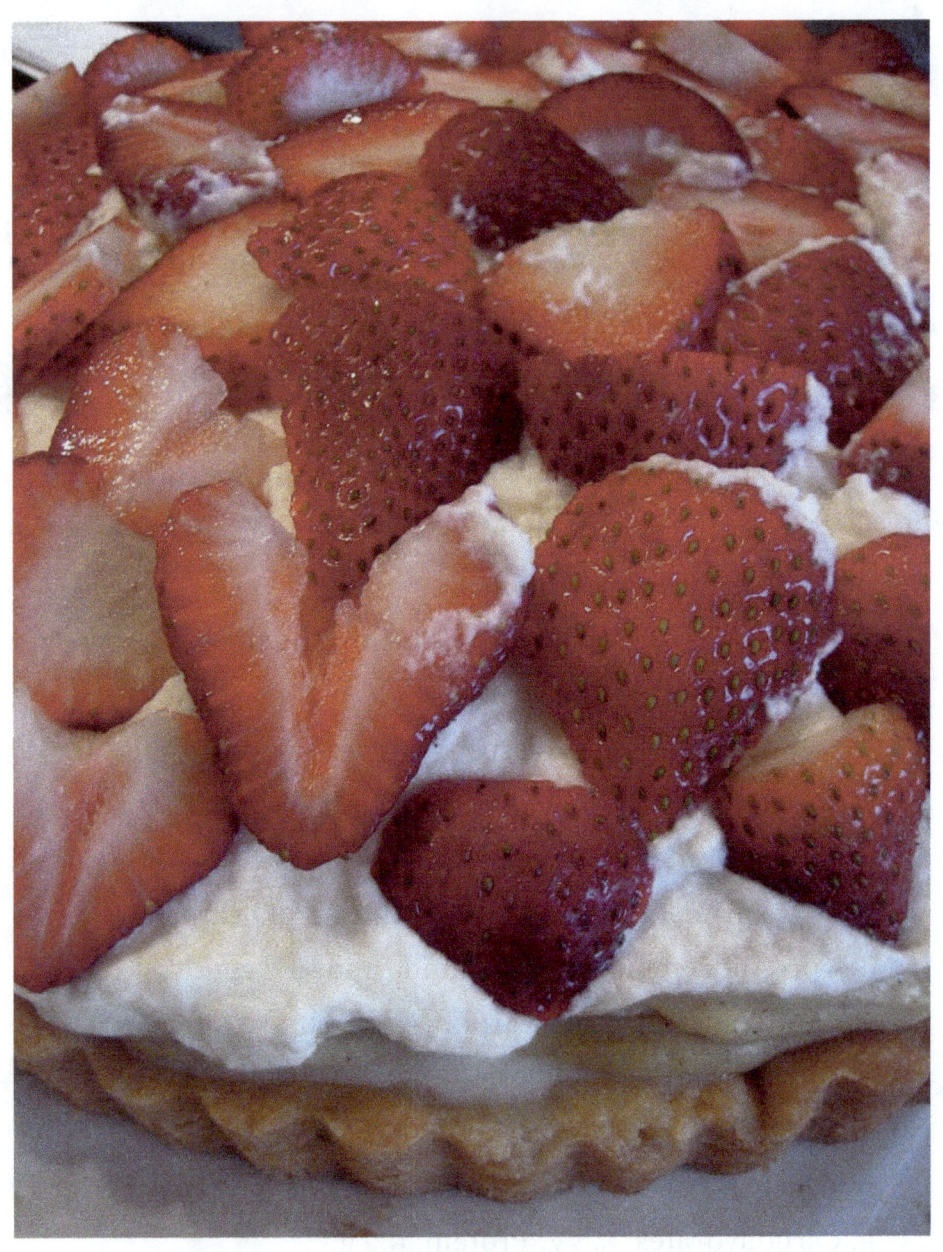

Strawberry Cream Pie

Servings: 3

Cooking Time: 2 Minutes

Ingredients:

- Shortbread Crust:
- 1 1/2 cups almond flour
- 1/4 cup powdered Swerve Sweetener
- 1/4 tsp salt
- 1/4 cup butter melted
- Strawberry Cream Filling:
- 1 cup heavy whipping cream
- 1 1/2 cups fresh strawberries, chopped
- 1/4 cup water
- 2 1/2 tsp gelatine, grass fed
- 1/2 cup powdered Swerve Sweetener
- 3/4 tsp vanilla essence
- whipped cream for serving

Directions:

1. Mix almond flour with salt and sweetener in a medium bowl.
2. Whisk in melted butter and mix well to form a coarse mixture.
3. Spread this mixture in a pie plate.

4. Spread the crust mixture into the plate and press it firmly.
5. Freeze this crust until the filling is prepared.
6. Strawberry Cream Filling:
7. Puree the strawberries in a blender or food processor with water.
8. Cook this puree with gelatine in a saucepan on low heat.
9. Bring it to a low simmer then turn off the heat. Allow it to cool for 20 minutes.
10. Beat cream with vanilla essence and sweetener in a suitable bowl.
11. Stir in strawberry mixture and mix well until smooth.
12. Spread this mixture into the frozen crust.
13. Refrigerate this pie for 3 hours.
14. Garnish with whipped cream and berries.
15. Serve.

Nutrition Info: Per Servings: Calories 321 Total Fat 12.9 g Saturated Fat 5.1 g Cholesterol 17 mg Total Carbs 8.1 g Sugar 1.8 g Fiber 0.4 g Sodium 28 mg Potassium 137 mg Protein 5.4 g

Delicious Custard Tarts

Servings: 8

Cooking Time: 30 Minutes

Ingredients:

- For crust:
- ¾ cup coconut flour
- 1 tbsp swerve
- 2 eggs
- ½ cup of coconut oil
- Pinch of salt
- For custard:
- 3 eggs
- ½ tsp nutmeg
- 5 tbsp swerve
- 1 ½ tsp vanilla
- 1 ¼ cup unsweetened almond milk

Directions:

1. For the crust: Preheat the oven to 400 F 200 C.
2. In a bowl, beat eggs, coconut oil, sweetener, and salt.
3. Add coconut flour and mix until dough is formed.
4. Add dough in the tart pan and spread evenly.
5. Prick dough with a knife.
6. Bake in preheated oven for 10 minutes.

7. For the custard: Heat almond milk and vanilla in a small pot until simmering.
8. Whisk together eggs and sweetener in a bowl. Slowly add almond milk and whisk constantly.
9. Strain custard well and pour into baked tart base.
10. Bake in the oven at 300 F for 30 minutes.
11. Sprinkle nutmeg on top and serve.

Nutrition Info: Per Servings: Net Carbs: 2.2g; Calories: 175; Total Fat: 17.2g; Saturated Fat: 9g Protein: 3.8g; Carbs: 2.9g; Fiber: 0.7g; Sugar: 0.4g; Fat 87% Protein 8% Carbs 5%

Butter Pie

Servings: 8

Cooking Time: 50 Minutes

Ingredients:

- For crust:
- 1 egg
- 14 cup butter, melted
- 3 tbsp erythritol
- 1 14 cup almond flour
- For filling:
- 1 egg
- 1 egg yolk
- 8 oz cream cheese, softened
- 1 cup butter, melted
- 12 cup erythritol

Directions:

1. Preheat the oven to 375 F 0 C.
2. Spray a 9-inch pie dish with cooking spray and set aside.
3. For the crust: In a large bowl, mix together all crust ingredients until well combined.
4. Transfer crust mixture into the prepared dish. Spread evenly and lightly press down with your fingers.
5. Bake in preheated oven for 7 minutes.

6. Remove from oven and set aside to cool completely.
7. For the filling: In a mixing bowl, add all filling ingredients and mix using an electric mixer until well combined.
8. Pour filling mixture into the crust and bake at 350 F 1 C for 35-40 minutes.
9. Remove from oven and set aside to cool completely.
10. Place in refrigerator for 1-2 hours.
11. Slice and serve.

Nutrition Info: Per Servings: Net Carbs: 2.8g; Calories: 476 Total Fat: 49.1g; Saturated Fat: 25.6g Protein: 7.9g; Carbs: 4.7g; Fiber: 1.9g; Sugar: 0.8g; Fat 92% Protein 6% Carbs 2%

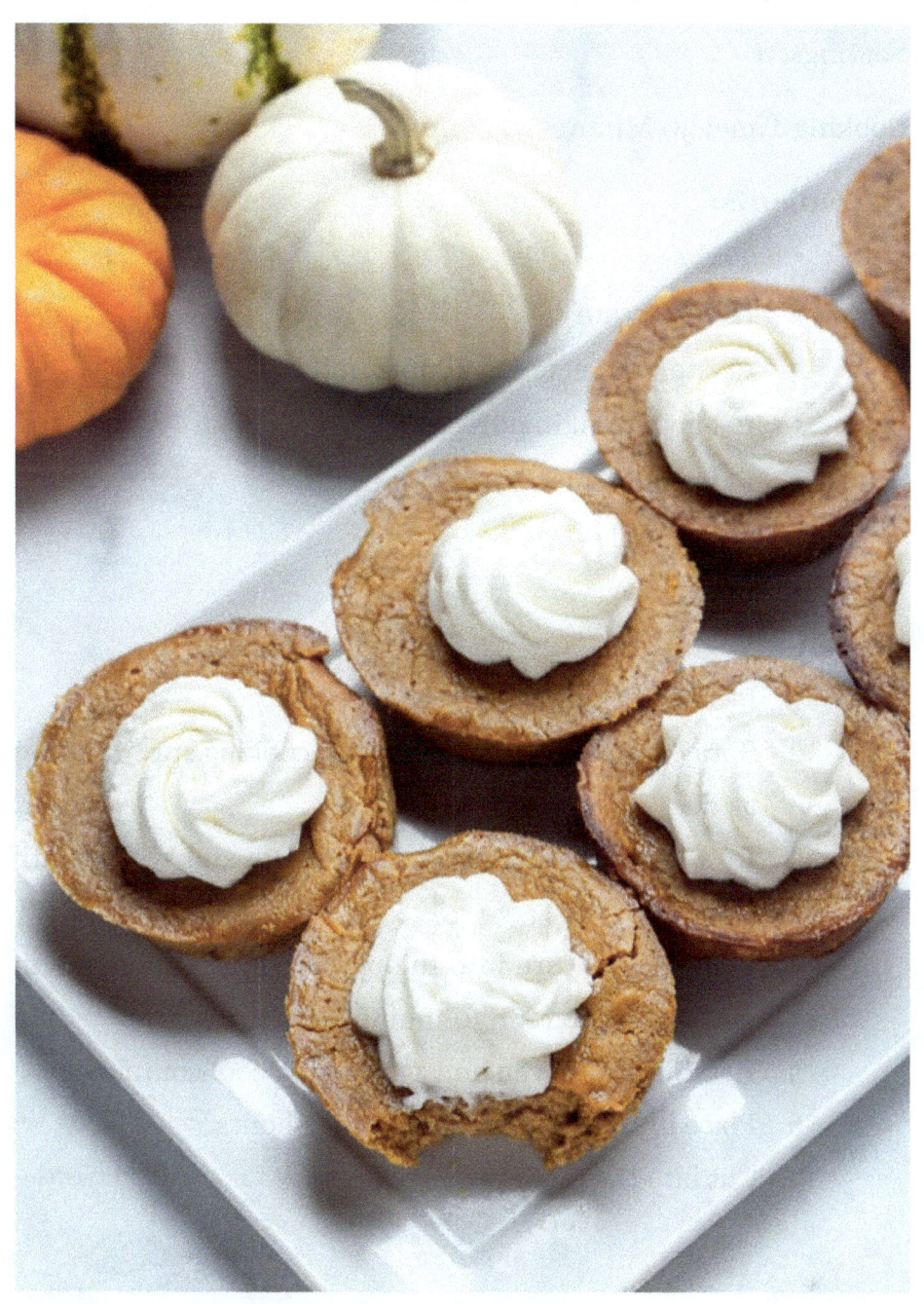

Crust-less Pumpkin Pie

Servings: 4

Cooking Time: 30 Minutes

Ingredients:

- 3 eggs
- 12 cup cream
- 12 cup unsweetened almond milk
- 12 cup pumpkin puree
- 12 tsp cinnamon
- 1 tsp vanilla
- 14 cup Swerve

Directions:

1. Preheat the oven to 350 F 0 C.
2. Spray a square baking dish with cooking spray and set aside.
3. In a large bowl, add all ingredients and whisk until smooth.
4. Pour pie mixture into the prepared dish and bake in preheated oven for 30 minutes.
5. Remove from oven and set aside to cool completely.
6. Place into the refrigerator for 1-2 hours.
7. Cut into the pieces and serve.

Nutrition Info: Per Servings: Net Carbs: 3.2g; Calories: ; Total Fat: 5.5g; Saturated Fat: 2.1g Protein: 4.9g; Carbs: 4.4g; Fiber: 1.2g; Sugar: 2g; Fat 60% Protein 25% Carbs 15%

Almond Meal Vanilla Tart

Servings: 4

Cooking Time: 25 Minutes

Ingredients:

- Crust
- 1 tablespoon swerve
- 6 teaspoons flaxseed meal
- 1/4 teaspoon nutmeg
- 1/2 oz. butter, unsalted, melted
- 6 tablespoons almond meal
- 1/2 egg
- Filling
- 1/2 vanilla bean
- 1 egg
- 1 egg yolk
- 1 1/4 tablespoon erythritol
- 3/4 cup whipping cream

Directions:

1. Let the oven preheat at 350 degrees F.
2. Mix everything or the crust in a suitable bowl.
3. Spread and press this mixture in a greased pie pan.
4. Bake this crust for 12 minutes in the preheated oven at 350 degrees F.

5. Once done, keep the crust at room temperature to cool.
6. Filling
7. Decrease the temperature of the oven to 320 degrees F.
8. Beat the vanilla seeds, swerve and egg yolks in eggs using a mixer.
9. Whisk in cream and stir well until smooth.
10. Pour this filling through a sieve and discard the vanilla seeds.
11. Spread this filling into the baked crust and return the pan to the oven.
12. Bake it again for 25 minutes approximately.
13. Allow the baked pie to cool at room temperature for 10 minutes.
14. Drizzle nutmeg on top then refrigerate for 30 minutes to chill.
15. Slice and enjoy.

Nutrition Info: Calories 215 ;Total Fat 20 g ;Saturated Fat 7 g ;Cholesterol 38 mg ;Sodium 12 mg ;Total Carbs 8 g ;Sugar 1 g ;Fiber 6 g ;Protein 5 g

Keto Lemon Curd Tarts With Blackberries

Servings: 6

Cooking Time: 15 Minutes

Ingredients:
- For lemon curd:
- ¼ cup lemon juice
- 2 egg yolks
- 1 small egg
- 6 tablespoons granulated monk fruit sweetener or erythritol
- 2 tablespoons butter or coconut oil, melted
- ½ tablespoon grated lemon zest
- For almond flour pie crust:
- ¾ cup blanched almond flour
- 2 tablespoons powdered erythritol
- 2 tablespoons cold, unsalted butter or refined coconut oil
- ¼ cup coconut flour
- 1 egg
- Other ingredients:
- ½ tablespoon sliced almonds
- 5 ounces blackberries or any other berries of your choice

- Powdered erythritol

Directions:
1. Add all the ingredients for crust into a bowl and mix well.
2. Grease a 9-inch pie pan with oil and line it with parchment paper. Place the dough in the pan and press it well on the bottom as well as the sides of the pan. Place the pan in the freezer for about 5-8 minutes.
3. Prick the crust with a fork in a few places.
4. Bake in a preheated oven 350° F for about 12 – 15 minutes or until light brown.
5. Remove from the oven and let it cool.
6. Meanwhile, make the lemon curd as follows: Add all the ingredients for lemon curd into a heatproof bowl. Place the bowl in a double boiler. Place the double boiler over medium heat.
7. Keep whisking until the mixture is thick.
8. Remove the bowl from the double boiler and pass the mixture through a fine wire mesh strainer placed over a bowl.
9. Stir the butter and let it cool completely.
10. Spread the lemon curd over the tart. Scatter blackberries and almonds on top. Finally sprinkle erythritol over the blackberries.
11. Cover with cling wrap. Chill until use. Preferably serve within 12 – 15 hours of preparing it.

12. Slice and serve.

Nutrition Info: Per Servings: Calories: 176 kcal, Fat: 15 g, Carbohydrates: 6.5 g, Protein: 5 g

Apple Tart

Servings: 10

Cooking Time: 55 Minutes

Ingredients:

- For crust:
- 2 cups almond flour
- 6 tbsp butter, melted
- 12 tsp cinnamon
- 13 cup erythritol
- For filling:
- 14 cup erythritol
- 3 cups apples, peeled, cored, and sliced
- 12 tsp cinnamon
- 14 cup butter
- 12 tsp lemon juice

Directions:

1. Preheat the oven to 375 F 0 C.
2. For the crust: In a bowl, mix together butter, cinnamon, swerve, and almond flour until it looks crumbly.
3. Transfer crust mixture into the 10-inch spring-form pan and spread evenly using your fingers.
4. Bake crust in preheated oven for 5 minutes.

5. For the filling: In a bowl, mix together apple slices and lemon juice.
6. Arrange apple slices evenly across the bottom of the baked crust in a circular shape.
7. Press apple slices down lightly.
8. In a small bowl, combine together butter, swerve, and cinnamon and microwave for 1 minute.
9. Whisk until smooth and pour over apple slices.
10. Bake tart for 30 minutes.
11. Remove from oven and lightly press down apple slices with a fork.
12. Turn heat to 350 F 180 C and bake for 20 minutes more.
13. Remove from the oven and set aside to cool completely.
14. Slice and serve.

Nutrition Info: Per Servings: Net Carbs: 3.7g; Calories: 236; Total Fat: 22.7g; Saturated Fat: 8.1g Protein: 5g; Carbs: 6.4g; Fiber: 2.7g; Sugar: 1.9g; Fat 86% Protein 8% Carbs 6%

Strawberry Vanilla Tart

Servings: 8

Cooking Time: 10 Minutes

Ingredients:

- Coconut crust:
- 1/2 cup coconut oil
- 3/4 cup 2 tablespoons coconut flour
- 2 eggs
- 1 teaspoon vanilla essence
- 1 teaspoon powdered sweetener
- Cream Filling:
- 1 cup mascarpone
- 2 eggs separated
- 1 teaspoon vanilla essence
- 1-2 tablespoons powdered sweetener
- 1 cup strawberries

Directions:

1. Crust:
2. Let your oven preheat at 350 degrees F.
3. Beat eggs in a suitable bowl then add rest of the ingredients.
4. Spread this dough in between two sheets of parchment paper.

5. Place this dough sheet in a greased pan and pierce holes in it using a fork.
6. Bake this crust for 10 minutes in the preheated oven.
7. Cream Filling:
8. Beat the egg whites in an electric mixer until frothy.
9. Stir in mascarpone cream, egg yolks, sweetener, and vanilla and beat for 2 minutes.
10. Spread this filling in the baked crust evenly.
11. Top the filling with the sweetener and strawberries.
12. Place the pie in the refrigerator for 30 minutes.
13. Slice and serve.

Nutrition Info: Calories 236 ;Total Fat 21.5 g ;Saturated Fat 15.2 g ;Cholesterol 54 mg ;Sodium 21 mg ;Total Carbs 7.6 g ;Sugar 1.4 g ;Fiber 3.8 g ;Protein 4.3 g

Cheesecake Tarts

Servings: 12

Cooking Time: 1 Hour And 30 Minutes

Ingredients:

- For the Crust:
- ¾ cup almond flour
- 3 tablespoons unsalted butter, melted
- For the Filling:
- ¼ teaspoon salt
- ¼ cup erythritol sweetener
- 1 tablespoon lemon juice
- 1 teaspoon vanilla extract, unsweetened
- 12-ounce cream cheese, softened
- 1 egg
- For the Toppings:
- ¼ cup blueberries
- ¼ cup strawberry jam, sugar-free

Directions:

1. Set oven to 350 degrees F and let preheat.
2. In the meantime, prepare the crust and for this stir together flour and butter until crumbly mixture comes together.

3. Take 12 cups muffin pan, line each tin with a paper cup, then add 1 to 2 teaspoons almond flour mixture and spread evenly on the bottom.
4. Place muffin pan into the oven and bake for 5 to 8 minutes or more until golden brown.
5. When done, transfer muffin pan on wire rack and let cool completely.
6. In the meantime, prepare the filling and for this, place cream cheese into the oven and beat with an electric beater at high speed until soft peaks form.
7. Beat in egg, sweetener, lemon juice, vanilla, and salt until mixed well and spoon the filling into cooled crusts.
8. Return muffin pan into the oven and bake for 20 minutes or until set.
9. When done, let muffins cool at room temperature for 10 minutes and then top each muffin with 1 teaspoon jam.
10. Top with berries, chill in refrigerator and serve.

Nutrition Info: Calories: 196 Cal, Carbs: 14 g, Fat: 16 g, Protein: 9 g, Fiber: 1.2 g.

Dark Chocolate Tart

Servings: 6

Cooking Time: 27 Minutes

Ingredients:

- Crust
- 6 tbsp coconut flour
- 2 tbsp erythritol
- 4 tbsp butter, melted
- 2 4-inch tart pans
- 1 large egg
- Filling
- 1 large egg
- 2 oz sugar free chocolate, shredded
- 1/2 cup heavy whipping cream
- 30 drops liquid stevia
- 1/4 cup erythritol powder
- 1 oz cream cheese

Directions:

1. Let your oven preheat at 350 degrees F.
2. Mix all the crust ingredients in a mixing bowl.
3. Divide this mixture into 4 tart pans and press it well.
4. Poke, some holes in the crust, then bake each for 12 minutes.
5. Allow these tart crusts to cool until the filling is ready.

6. Warm the cream up in a saucepan then pour it into a jar.
7. Add chopped chocolate and blend well using a hand blender.
8. Stir in stevia, erythritol, egg and cream cheese. Blend well until smooth.
9. Divide this filling into the baked crusts and return them to the oven.
10. Bake them for 15 minutes at 325 degrees F.
11. Allow them to cool then refrigerate for 2 hours.
12. Serve.

Nutrition Info: Per Servings: Calories 175 Total Fat 16 g Saturated Fat 2.1 g Cholesterol 0 mg Total Carbs 2.8 g Sugar 1.8 g Fiber 0.4 g Sodium 8 mg Potassium 81 mg Protein 9 g

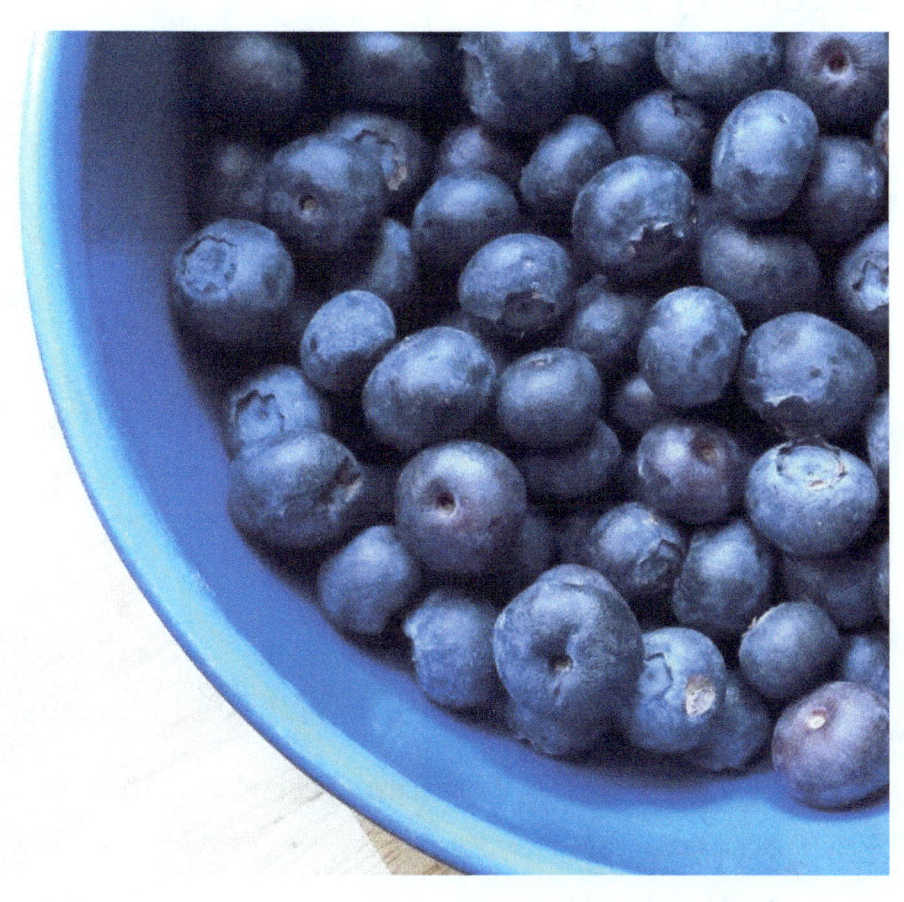

Blueberry Lemon

Servings: 4

Cooking Time: 1 Hour

Ingredients:

- For the crust:
- 1/4tsp. monk fruit sweetener
- 2 tbsp. coconut oil, melted
- 1/4 cup coconut flour
- 2 1/2 cups pecan pieces, raw
- 1/8tsp. salt
- 2 tbsp. almond butter, smooth
- For the filling:
- 3/4 cup lemon juice
- 12 tbsp. butter, unsalted and cubed
- 4 large eggs
- 1/4 cup lemon zest
- 2 tsp. monk fruit sweetener
- 1/8tsp. salt
- For the topping:
- 2 cups blueberries

Directions:

1. Crust:
2. Liberally butter four 4 3 /4-inch tart pans or cover with baking paper.

3. Use a food blender to combine the coconut flour, coconut oil, and almond butter for 2 minutes on high.
4. Add the monk fruit, pecan pieces, and salt until crumbly. Dividing the batter into equal parts, transfer them to the tart pans. Evenly compress the crust by hand. Begin with the sides of the pan with the middle being pressed last. Put in the refrigerator to set.
5. Filling:
6. In a regular dish, blend together the sweetener and lemon zest and stir with a large spoon.
7. Heat a medium saucepan halfway filled with water on low/medium.
8. In a heatproof big dish, pour in the lemon juice, lemon zest, and eggs. Place the bowl on top of the saucepan.
9. Wait until the water starts to simmer. Then whisk the ingredients until they thicken for approximately 10 minutes.
10. Using a fine-mesh strainer, pour and press the curd into a blender.
11. After adding the salt, turn the blender on the low setting. Start adding the cubes of butter 3 pieces at a time and repeat until all the butter is blended. Move the tart pans to the counter and pour the filling inside the crusts.

12. Put the tart pans back into the refrigerator for 20 minutes to set and cool. Shake the blueberries over the tarts and serve.
13. Tricks and Tips:
14. If you prefer your crust baked, put the tart pans in the stove at 375° Fahrenheit. Heat the crusts for 13 minutes. Then follow steps 7 through 9.
15. If not eating the curd right away, pour into a container with plastic wrap tightly pressed on the top. Keep in the fridge, and the curd will stay fresh for 1 week.

Nutrition Info: 8 grams ;Net Carbs: 4.9 grams ;Fat: 20 grams ;Calories: 21

Lemon Meringue Pie

Servings: 6

Cooking Time: 4 Hours And 30 Minutes

Ingredients:

- For the Crust:
- ½ cup almond flour
- ½ cup coconut flour
- 2 tablespoons Swerve sweetener
- 1 teaspoon vanilla extract, unsweetened
- 2 teaspoons arrowroot
- ½ cup unsalted butter, cut in small cubes
- 2 eggs
- For the Filling:
- 1 tablespoon arrowroot
- ¼ teaspoon salt
- 1 ¼ cups Swerve sugar
- 1 envelope of gelatin
- 3 tablespoons unsalted butter
- 2 teaspoons grated lemon zest
- ½ cup lemon juice
- 1 ¼ cup water
- 4 egg yolks, beaten
- For the Meringue:
- ½ cup Swerve sugar

- 4 egg whites
- ½ teaspoon cream of tartar

Directions:
1. Set oven to 350 degrees F and let preheat.
2. In the meantime, place all the ingredients for crust in a food processor and pulse for 10 to 1minutes or until crumbly.
3. Take a 9-inch pie dish, line with parchment paper, then spoon in prepared crust mixture and spread and press down using hands and then with a back of a spoon.
4. Place pie dish into the oven and bake for 10 to 12 minutes or until nicely brown.
5. In the meantime, prepare the filling and for this, place a small saucepan over medium heat, and add salt, sweetener, gelatin, and water.
6. Stir well until gelatin dissolves and bring the mixture to boil.
7. Then boil for 1 minute, slowly pour in egg yolks and continue cooking until thickened.
8. Whisk in lemon juice and zest, and butter, then remove the pan from heat and set aside.
9. Prepare meringue and for this, place egg whites in a bowl and whip at low speed until foamy.
10. Then slowly whisk in sugar until stiff peaks form.

11. When pie crust is done, spoon filling into it and top completely with prepared meringue.
12. Return pie into the oven and bake for 30 minutes or until meringue is lightly browned.
13. When done, cool pie at room temperature for 1 hour and then in the refrigerator for 3 hours.
14. Slice and serve.

Nutrition Info: Calories: 217 Cal, Carbs: 9 g, Fat: 19 g, Protein: 7 g, Fiber: 3 g.

Grasshopper Pie

Servings: 5

Cooking Time: 5 Minutes

Ingredients:

- For brownie crust:
- ¾ cup + 2 tablespoons walnuts
- 2 tablespoons coconut oil
- A pinch stevia or monk fruit sweetener
- For mint cream filling:
- 1 cup raw cashews, soaked in hot water for 2 hours, drained, rinsed
- ¼ cup coconut milk
- A large pinch stevia or monk fruit sweetener
- ½ cup tightly packed fresh baby spinach
- 1/3 cup melted coconut oil
- 1 teaspoon mint extract
- ½ tablespoon vanilla
- A pinch Himalayan pink salt
- To garnish:
- A few cacao nibs

Directions:

1. For crust: Add all the ingredients for crust into the food processor bowl. Fix the "S" blade and process until dough is formed. Process until dough is formed.

It should be sticky dough. Sprinkle a little water if necessary while processing.
2. Line a 6-inch pie pan with parchment paper. Place the dough in the pan and press it well on the bottom and sides of the pan.
3. For the filling: Dry the cashews with paper towels and add into the food processor bowl.
4. Add spinach and process until chopped into smaller pieces.
5. Add the rest of the ingredients and process until well combined and smooth.
6. Spread the filling over the crust. Cover the pan with cling wrap and freeze for about 2 hours.
7. Scatter cocoa nibs on top if using.
8. Slice and serve.

Nutrition Info: Per Servings: Calories: 435.6 kcal, Fat: 42.2 g, Carbohydrates: 2 g, Protein: 7 g

Lemon Pie

Servings: 8

Cooking Time: 15 Minutes

Ingredients:

- For crust:
- 1 cup pecans, chopped
- 1 tsp swerve
- 2 tbsp butter, melted
- For filling:
- 1 tsp vanilla
- 1 1⁄2 cup heavy whipping cream
- 8 oz cream cheese, softened
- 2⁄3 cup Swerve
- 1⁄4 cup fresh lemon juice
- 1 tbsp lemon zest

Directions:

1. Preheat the oven to 350 F 0 C.
2. Add pecans into the food processor and process until pecans crush finely.
3. Add swerve and butter into the crushed pecans and mix until well combined.
4. Spray pie pan with cooking spray.
5. Add crust mixture into the prepared pan.

6. Spread evenly and lightly press down with your fingers.
7. Bake in preheated oven for 10 minutes.
8. Remove from oven and set aside to cool completely.
9. For the filling: In a large bowl, beat whipping cream until stiff peaks forms.
10. Add vanilla, swerve, and cream cheese and beat until smooth.
11. Add lemon zest and lemon juice and beat until just combined.
12. Pour filling mixture into the baked crust and spread evenly.
13. Place in refrigerator for 1-2 hours.
14. Slice and serve.

Nutrition Info: Per Servings: Net Carbs: 2.3g; Calories: 311 Total Fat: 32.2g; Saturated Fat: 14.3g Protein: 4.2g; Carbs: 3.9g; Fiber: 1.6g; Sugar: 0.9g; Fat 93% Protein 5% Carbs 2%

Quick & Simple Strawberry Tart

Servings: 10

Cooking Time: 22 Minutes

Ingredients:

- 5 egg whites
- ½ cup butter, melted
- 1 tsp baking powder
- 1 tsp vanilla
- 1 lemon zest, grated
- 1 ½ cup almond flour
- 13 cup xylitol

Directions:

1. Preheat the oven to 375 F 0 C.
2. Spray the tart pan with cooking spray and set aside.
3. In a bowl, whisk egg whites until foamy.
4. Add sweetener and whisk until soft peaks form.
5. Add remaining ingredients except for strawberries and fold until well combined.
6. Pour mixture into the prepared tart pan and top with sliced strawberries.
7. Bake in preheated oven for 20-22 minutes.
8. Serve and enjoy.

Nutrition Info: Per Servings: Net Carbs: 3.; Calories: 195; Total Fat: 17.7g; Saturated Fat: 6.4g Protein: 5.6g; Carbs: 5.9g; Fiber: 2g; Sugar: 0.9g; Fat 81% Protein 11% Carbs 8%

Easy Lemon Pie

Servings: 8

Cooking Time: 45 Minutes

Ingredients:

- 3 eggs
- 3 lemon juice
- 1 lemon zest, grated
- 4 oz erythritol
- 5.5 oz almond flour
- 3.5 oz butter, melted
- Salt

Directions:

1. Preheat the oven to 350 F 0 C.
2. In a bowl, mix together butter, 1 oz sweetener, 3 oz almond flour, and salt.
3. Transfer the dough in a pie dish and spread evenly and bake for 20 minutes.
4. In a separate bowl, mix together eggs, lemon juice, lemon zest, remaining flour, sweetener, and salt.
5. Pour egg mixture on prepared crust and bake for 2minutes more.
6. Allow to cool completely.
7. Slice and serve.

Nutrition Info: Per Servings: Net Carbs: 3.0g; Calories: 229; Total Fat: 21.5g; Saturated Fat: 7.7g Protein: 6.5g; Carbs: 5.3g; Fiber: 2.3g; Sugar: 1.4g; Fat % Protein 11% Carbs 5%

Chocolate Keto Pudding

Servings: 8

Cooking Time: 20 Minutes

Ingredients:

- 2 cups heavy cream
- 2/3 cup Truvia or other sugar substitute
- 2 extra-large eggs
- 2 teaspoons vanilla extract
- 2 cups unsweetened almond milk
- ½ cup unsweetened cocoa powder
- 2 teaspoons xanthan gum
- Whipped cream to serve

Directions:

1. Add heavy cream, cocoa, xanthan gum, milk, eggs and truvia into a saucepan.
2. Place the saucepan over medium-low heat. Stir frequently until the mixture is thick and can coat the back of the spoon. Do not boil the mixture. Turn off the heat and add vanilla. Mix well.
3. Transfer into a serving bowl. Cover with cling wrap and chill until use.
4. Serve in bowls topped with whipped cream.

Nutrition Info: Per Servings: Calories: 239 kcal, Fat: 22.6 g, Carbohydrates: 6 g, Protein: 5.6 g

Fruit And Cheese

Servings: 12

Cooking Time: 2 Hours 15 Minutes

Ingredients:

- 12 prepared tart crusts, (see tricks and tips below)
- 1/3 cup lemon juice
- 14 oz. condensed milk, sweetened
- 1 tsp. lemon zest
- 8 oz. cream cheese, softened
- 1/4 cup crab apple jelly, melted
- 3 tbsp. coconut, toasted
- 12 pineapple chunks
- 1 tsp. almond extract
- 12 blackberries
- 4 large strawberries, sliced
- 1 tsp. vanilla extract, sugar-free

Directions:

1. Place the prepared tart crusts on two baking paper lined cookie sheets. You can also use a non-stick baking mat.
2. In a regular dish, blend together the cream cheese and condensed milk until soft. Combine the lemon zest and lemon juice, stirring with a rubber scraper. Then

blend the almond extract and vanilla extract until smooth.
3. Sprinkle 4 teaspoons of toasted coconut into each tart crust and pour the cream cheese on top.
4. Put the tarts into the refrigerator for 2 hours to harden.
5. Just before serving, use a small saucepan on low heat to melt the crab apple jelly.
6. Remove the tarts and garnish with a strawberry slice, pineapple chunk, and a blackberry. Drizzle the crab apple jelly on top of the fruit and serve.
7. Tricks and Tips:
8. If you prefer your crust to be homemade, follow the baked tart crust steps in the Blueberry Lemon Tart recipe.

Nutrition Info: 5 grams ;Net Carbs: 5 grams ;Fat: 16 grams ;Calories: 187

Low Carb Lemon Tart

Servings: 6

Cooking Time: 20 Minutes

Ingredients:

- For crust:
- ¼ cup coconut flour
- ¾ cup almond flour
- A small pinch salt
- 1/8 teaspoon vanilla extract
- 1 ½ tablespoons butter, melted
- ¼ teaspoon xanthan gum (optional)
- 1 small egg
- 2 tablespoons powdered erythritol or Swerve sweetener
- For lemon curd:
- ¼ cup lemon juice
- 2 egg yolks
- 1 small egg
- 6 tablespoons granulated monk fruit sweetener or erythritol
- 2 tablespoons butter or coconut oil, melted
- ½ tablespoon grated lemon zest

Directions:

1. Add the flours, oil, egg, vanilla, butter, xanthan gum, salt and sweetener into a food processor bowl. Fix the "S" blade and process until dough is formed. It will be crumbly.
2. Line a 6-inch pie pan with parchment paper. Place the dough in the pan and press it well on the bottom as well as the sides of the pan. Place the pan in the freezer for about – 30 minutes.
3. Prick the crust with a fork in a few places.
4. Bake in a preheated oven 320° F for about 15 – 20 minutes or until golden brown.
5. Add all the ingredients for lemon curd into a heatproof bowl. Place the bowl in a double boiler. Place the double boiler over medium heat.
6. Keep whisking until the mixture is thick.
7. Remove the bowl from the double boiler and pass the mixture through a fine wire mesh strainer placed over a bowl.
8. Stir in butter and let it cool completely.
9. Spread the lemon curd over the tart.
10. Cover with cling wrap. Chill until served. Preferably serve within 12 – 15 hours of preparing the tart.

Nutrition Info: Per Servings: Calories: 203 kcal, Fat: 17.8 g, Carbohydrates: 6 g, Protein: 6 g

Cheesecake Jam Tarts

Servings: 8

Cooking Time: 28 Minutes

Ingredients:

- Crust
- 3 tablespoons butter, melted
- ¾ cup almond flour
- Filling
- 12 oz. cream cheese,
- 1 egg
- ¼ cup erythritol
- 1 teaspoon vanilla essence
- 1 tablespoon fresh lemon juice
- ¼ teaspoon salt
- Toppings
- ¼ cup sugar-free strawberry jam
- ¼ cup blueberries

Directions:

1. Let your oven preheat at
2. Preheat your oven to 350 degrees F.
3. Mix almond flour with butter in a bowl.
4. Divide this mixture into the muffin tin and press it firmly.
5. Bake for 8 minutes until golden brown.

6. Meanwhile, beat cream cheese in an electric mixture along with 1 egg.
7. Beat in erythritol, vanilla essence, salt, and lemon juice and mix well.
8. Divide this filling into the muffin crust.
9. Bake the mini tarts for 20 minutes, then allow it to cool
10. Top with jam and blueberries.
11. Refrigerate overnight then Serve.

Nutrition Info: Calories 175 ;Total Fat 16 g ;Saturated Fat 2.1 g ;Cholesterol 0 mg ;Sodium 8 mg ;Total Carbs 2.8 g ;Sugar 1.8 g ;Fiber 0.4 g ;Protein 9 g

Mock Apple Pie

Servings: 8

Cooking Time: 40 Minutes

Ingredients:

- For crust:
- ¼ cup butter, melted (measure first and then melt)
- 6 tablespoons coconut flour
- ½ tablespoon whole psyllium husks
- ¾ cup almond flour
- 2 eggs
- ¼ teaspoon salt
- For filling:
- 5 small chayote squash, peeled, sliced
- ¾ teaspoon ground cinnamon
- A pinch ground nutmeg
- 1/8 teaspoon ground ginger
- ½ tablespoon xanthan gum
- ½ tablespoon lemon juice
- 3 tablespoons butter, cut into pieces
- 6 tablespoons Swerve or erythritol + extra to sprinkle
- 1 teaspoon apple extract (optional)
- 1 small egg, beaten, to brush onto top crust

Directions:

1. To make crust: Add all the ingredients for crust into a bowl and mix well to form into dough.
2. Divide into equal portions and shape into balls.
3. Take a 6-inch pie pan. Place the dough in it. Press it well onto the bottom as well as the sides of the pan. Set aside the other ball of dough.
4. Place chayote slices in a saucepan. Cover with water. Place saucepan over medium heat. Cook until chayote is tender. Drain the water from the saucepan.
5. Add the chayote back into the saucepan. Add the rest of the ingredients for the filling except butter and mix well.
6. Spread the chayote mixture on the crust. Place butter pieces all over the filling.
7. Roll the other ball of dough and place over the filling. Press the edges of both the crusts together to seal.
8. Make a few small slits in the top crust for the steam to escape. Lightly brush beaten egg all over the top crust.
9. Sprinkle some sweetener all over the crust if desired.
10. Bake in a preheated oven at 350° F for around 30 minutes or until golden brown on top.
11. Cool slightly. Cut into 8 equal slices and serve.

Nutrition Info: per Servings: Calories: 426.3 kcal, Fat: 33.5 g, Carbohydrates: 13 g, Protein: 15.1 g

Strawberry Pie With Gelatin

Servings: 6

Cooking Time: 20 Minutes

Ingredients:
- 1 coconut pie crust – refer to the first recipe in this chapter
- ½ cup powdered erythritol or Swerve
- ¼ cup water
- 1 pound strawberries, fresh or frozen
- 1 ½ tablespoons grass-fed gelatin
- 1 tablespoon lemon juice
- To serve:
- Whipped cream
- Fresh strawberry slices

Directions:
1. Have your pie crust ready.
2. Add strawberries and sweetener into a saucepan. Place the saucepan over medium heat.
3. Cook until soft stirring occasionally.
4. Meanwhile, add water, gelatin and lemon juice into a bowl and whisk well. Let it rest for 2-3 minutes.
5. Pour the gelatin mixture into the saucepan of strawberries. Whisk well. Let it cook for 1-2 minutes

until gelatin is dissolved. Turn off the heat and let the mix cool for about 20 minutes.
6. Spread the strawberries over the pie crust. Let it cool completely.
7. Chill for 8-9 hours.
8. Top with strawberry slices and cream. Cut into slices and serve.

Nutrition Info: Per Servings: Calories: 30.5 kcal, Fat: 5.2 g, Carbohydrates: 1.8 g, Protein: 2 g

Pumpkin Pie

Servings: 4

Cooking Time: 15 Minutes

Ingredients:

- For crust:
- 1 ½ cups coconut flakes, unsweetened
- 4 tablespoons Brain octane oil or ½ tablespoon melted ghee or coconut oil
- 1 tablespoon coconut cream
- ¼ - ½ tablespoon Swerve or erythritol
- For pumpkin filling:
- 1 ½ tablespoons coconut oil or ghee or butter, melted
- 1 teaspoon CollaGelatin
- 7.5 ounces steamed pumpkin or canned solid pumpkin puree
- 1 teaspoon vanilla extract
- Pinch of ground cloves or cardamom
- ¼ cup coconut cream
- 2 tablespoons water
- 1 ½ teaspoons ground Ceylon cinnamon
- A pinch salt
- To serve:
- Keto vanilla ice cream or whipped coconut cream.

Directions:

1. Add coconut into the food processor bowl. Process until very fine. Add the rest of the ingredients for crust and process until dough is formed.
2. Line a 6-inch pie pan with parchment paper. Place the dough in the pan and press it well on the bottom as well as the sides of the pan. Place the pan in the freezer for about – 30 minutes.
3. Meanwhile, add CollaGelatin and water in a bowl and stir. Set aside for 5-8 minutes.
4. Place a saucepan with coconut cream over low heat. Add CollaGelatin mixture. Stir frequently until it dissolves completely. Turn off the heat.
5. Transfer into a blender. Add the rest of the ingredients for the filling and blend until smooth.
6. Spread the filling over the crust. Cover the pan with cling wrap and freeze for about 2 hours.
7. Serve with suggested serving options.

Nutrition Info: Per Servings: Calories: 445 kcal, Fat: 46 g, Carbohydrates: 12.3 g, Protein: 7.5 g

Strawberry Tart

Servings: 10

Cooking Time: 25 Minutes

Ingredients:

- 1 egg
- 14 cup butter, melted
- 2 cups almond flour
- 1 tsp vanilla
- 14 cup Swerve
- For filling:
- 4 oz cream cheese
- 1 cup fresh strawberries, sliced
- 2 tbsp heavy cream
- 6 tbsp swerve
- 8 oz mascarpone cheese
- 12 tsp xanthan gum
- 1 tsp vanilla

Directions:

1. Preheat the oven to 350 F 0 C.
2. Spray the tart pan with cooking spray and set aside.
3. For the crust: Add almond flour, vanilla, swerve, egg, and butter into the food processor and process until it forms into a dough.
4. Transfer dough into the prepared tart pan.

5. Spread dough evenly and lightly press down with your fingers.
6. Prick crust dough with a knife and cover with parchment paper and dried beans.
7. Bake in preheated oven for 20 minutes.
8. Remove from oven and set aside to cool completely.
9. For the filling: Add strawberries, heavy cream, swerve, vanilla, cream cheese, and mascarpone cheese into the food processor and process until smooth and creamy.
10. Add xanthan gum and stir well.
11. Pour filling mixture into baked crust and spread evenly.
12. Place into the refrigerator for 1-2 hours.
13. Slices and serve.

Nutrition Info: Per Servings: Net Carbs: 6.4g; Calories: 277 Total Fat: 24.3g; Saturated Fat: 8.9g Protein: 9g; Carbs: 9.3g; Fiber: 2.9g; Sugar: 1.7g; Fat 79% Protein 12% Carbs 9%

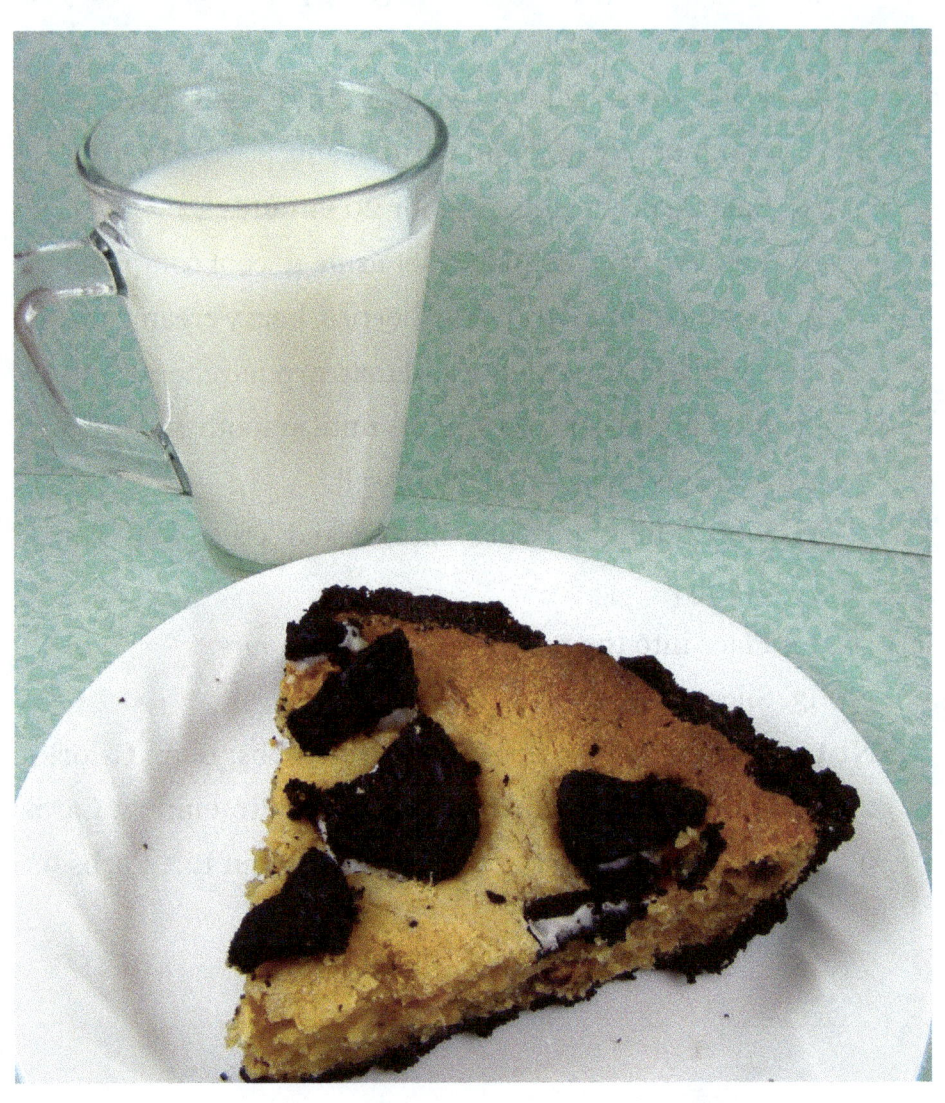

Cookie Pie

Servings: 4

Cooking Time: 15 Minutes

Ingredients:

- 0.5 ounce coconut flour
- 2 ounces almond flour
- 2 teaspoons golden flax meal
- A pinch salt
- 1/8 teaspoon baking powder
- 3 ounces butter or coconut butter, at room temperature
- ½ teaspoon vanilla extract
- 1.5 ounces chopped pecans
- 4-6 tablespoons monk fruit sweetener
- 2 ounces stevia sweetened dark chocolate bar, chopped or dark chocolate chips
- A large pinch of flaky sea salt, to garnish

Directions:

1. Place a skillet over medium heat. Add almond flour and toast until golden brown and aromatic. Remove on a plate and let it cool completely.
2. Take 4 small pie pans (4 inches each) and grease with butter or oil. You can use ramekins as well.

3. Add almond flour, flaxseed meal, coconut flour, salt and baking powder into a bowl and stir well.
4. Add butter into a mixing bowl. Beat with an electric hand mixer until creamy.
5. Add vanilla and beat until well combined.
6. Set the mixer on low speed and add flour mixture, a little at a time (about ¼) and beat until just combined each time.
7. Add chocolate and pecan bits and fold gently. Divide the dough into the pie pans. Press it well into the pans. Freeze for 20 minutes.
8. Bake in a preheated oven at 360° F for around 15 – 1minutes until it starts to become brown.
9. Remove from the oven and let it cool for 15 minutes. Serve the cookie pie with bowls, since it tends to stick to the pan.

Nutrition Info: Per Servings: Calories: 306.7 kcal, Fat: 26.5 g, Carbohydrates: 14 g, Protein: 4.3 g

Low Carb Vanilla Pudding

Servings: 12

Cooking Time: 20 Minutes

Ingredients:

- 2 cups heavy cream
- 2/3 cup granulated Swerve or Sukrin:1 (or other sugar-free, natural sweetener)
- 1/8 teaspoon salt
- 6 large egg yolks
- 4 eggs
- 1 cup almond milk
- 2 tablespoons cornstarch
- 2 teaspoons vanilla extract
- 4 tablespoons butter
- ½ teaspoon stevia Glycerite
- 1 ½ teaspoons gelatin powder, soaked in 2 tablespoons water for 5 minutes

Directions:

1. Add cream and almond milk into a pot. Place the pot over medium heat. Let simmer.
2. Add sweetener, salt and cornstarch into a bowl and stir.

3. Whisk in the yolks. Add eggs and whisk well. Pour the simmering mixture slowly into the bowl of eggs and whisk constantly until well combined.
4. Pour the mixture into the pot. Place the pot back over medium-low heat.
5. Keep whisking the mixture until it thickens slightly. Lower the heat to low heat and continue whisking for a couple of minutes.
6. Turn off the heat and continue whisking for another minute.
7. Pass the mixture through a fine wire mesh strainer placed over a bowl.
8. Add vanilla, butter and stevia Glycerite and whisk well. Add more sweetener if desired.
9. Add gelatin mixture and whisk well.
10. Cover the bowl with cling wrap. The wrap should touch the top of the pudding. This is to prevent forming a film on top of the pudding.
11. Refrigerate for 8-10 hours.
12. Remove from the refrigerator and whip the pudding with an electric hand mixer.
13. Divide into bowls and serve.

Nutrition Info: Per Servings: Calories: 222 kcal, Fat: 20.9 g, Carbohydrates: 4.1 g, Protein: 2.4 g

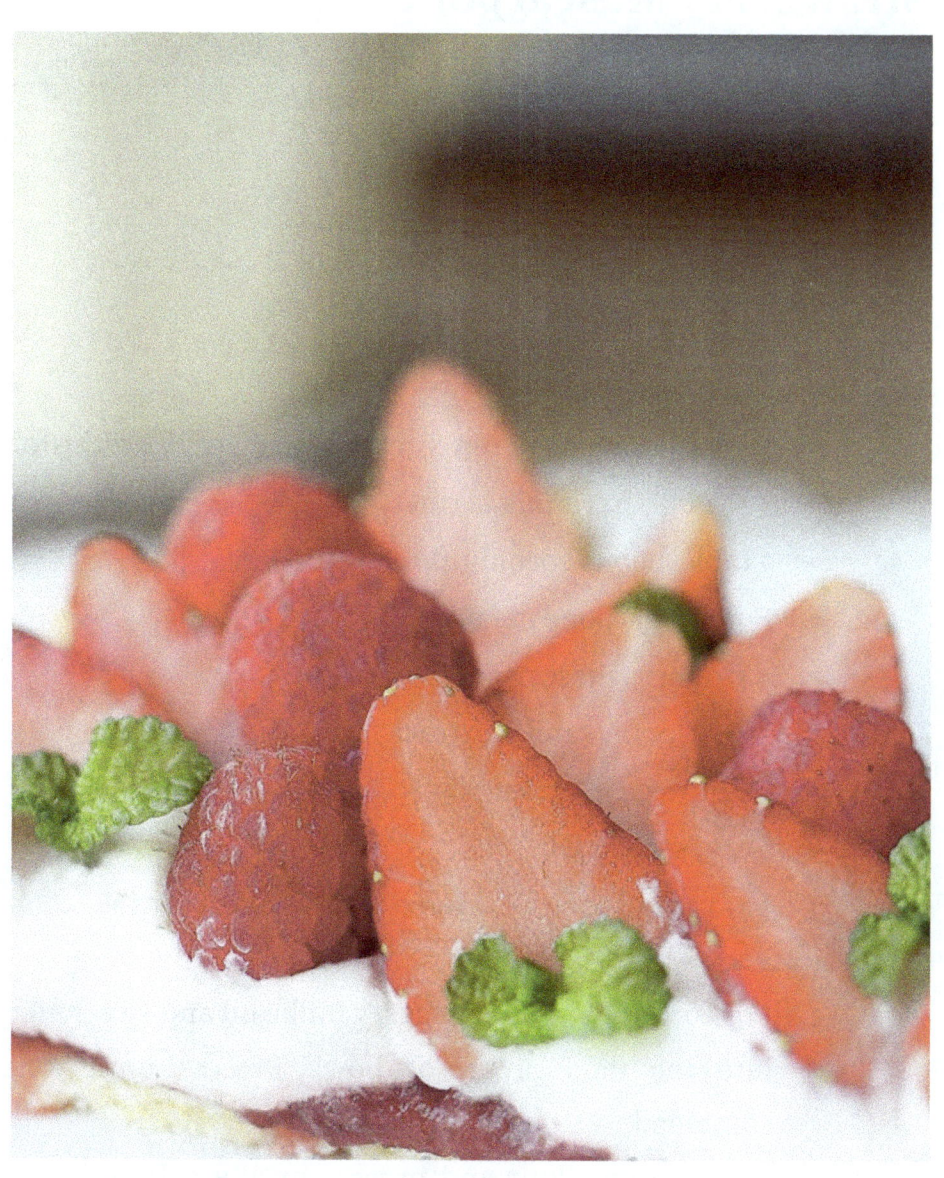

Strawberry Mascarpone Tart

Servings: 6

Cooking Time: 10 Minutes

Ingredients:

- For coconut base:
- ¼ cup coconut oil
- 1 egg
- ½ teaspoon powdered Swerve sweetener or erythritol
- ½ teaspoon vanilla extract
- 7 tablespoons coconut flour
- For mascarpone cream:
- 4.5 ounces mascarpone
- ½ teaspoon vanilla extract
- ½ cup strawberries
- 1 egg, separated
- ½ -1 tablespoon powdered Swerve or erythritol

Directions:

1. For coconut base: Add eggs, vanilla, oil and sweetener into the food processor bowl. Process until well combined.
2. Add coconut flour and process until a soft dough is formed.
3. Add more flour if necessary. Place the dough in the refrigerator for 10 – 15 minutes.

4. Line a 6-inch pie pan with parchment paper. Place the dough in the pan and press it well on the bottom as well as the sides of the pan. Place the pan in the freezer for about 20 – 30 minutes.
5. Prick the crust with a fork in a few places.
6. Bake in a preheated oven 350° F for about 15 – 20 minutes or until light brown.
7. For the filling: Beat the whites with an electric hand mixer until stiff peaks are formed.
8. Add yolks, mascarpone, sweetener and vanilla into a mixing bowl and whisk until well combined.
9. Add whites and fold gently. Spread the filling over the crust.
10. Chill for a couple of hours or until it sets.
11. Garnish with strawberry slices.
12. Slice and serve.

Nutrition Info: Per Servings: Calories: 118 kcal, Fat: 10 g, Carbohydrates: 5.7 g, Protein: 3.5 g

Key Lime Pie

Servings: 5

Cooking Time: 5-7 Minutes

Ingredients:

- For keto graham cracker crust:
- 3.5 ounces almond flour
- ½ teaspoon ground cinnamon
- 1 ounce butter, melted
- 2 -4 tablespoons Swerve sweetener or xylitol
- 1/8 teaspoon kosher salt
- For key lime filling:
- 7 ounces avocadoes, peeled, pitted, chopped
- 4.5 ounces coconut cream, chilled
- 2 tablespoons fresh key lime juice or to taste
- 1 tablespoon freshly grated key lime zest
- 1/8 teaspoon kosher salt or to taste
- 3-4 tablespoons powdered xylitol or Swerve or more to taste

Directions:

1. For keto graham cracker crust: Place a skillet over medium heat. Add almond flour and toast until golden in color and aromatic. Turn off the heat and add into a bowl. Let it cool for a few minutes.

2. Add Swerve, salt and cinnamon and stir. Stir in butter and mix until crumbly.
3. Divide into a 6-inch pie pan. Press it onto the bottom of the pan. Cool completely
4. Freeze for 10 – 20 minutes.
5. For key lime filling: Add all the ingredients for filling into a blender and blend until smooth. Taste and adjust the sweetener and salt if desired.
6. Spoon over the crust. Chill for 8-9 hours or freeze for 1-2 hours.
7. The pie can store for 3 to 4 days in the refrigerator.
8. Slice and serve.

Nutrition Info: Per Servings: Calories: 216.8 kcal, Fat: 21 g, Carbohydrates: 6.4 g, Protein: 3.6 g

Mascarpone Tart

Servings: 10

Cooking Time: 20 Minutes

Ingredients:
- For crust:
- 1 egg
- 14 cup butter, melted
- 2 cups almond flour
- 12 tsp vanilla
- 14 cup Swerve
- For filling:
- 6 oz mascarpone cheese
- 2 tbsp heavy cream
- 14 cup Swerve
- 34 cup lemon curd

Directions:
1. Spray the tart pan with cooking spray and set aside.
2. Preheat the oven to 350 F 180 C.
3. Add almond flour, vanilla, swerve, egg, and butter into the food processor and process until it forms a dough.
4. Add the dough into the prepared tart pan and spread out evenly.
5. Prick the crust with a fork and cover with parchment paper and dried beans.

6. Bake for 15 minutes.
7. Remove from oven and set aside to cool completely.
8. Add lemon curd, heavy cream, swerve, and mascarpone into the food processor and process until smooth and creamy.
9. Pour filling mixture into the baked crust and spread evenly.
10. Place in refrigerator for 2 hours.
11. Slice and serve.

Nutrition Info: Per Servings: Net Carbs: 5.6g; Calories: 174 Total Fat: 17.4g; Saturated Fat: 8.4g Protein: 3.1g; Carbs: 6.2g; Fiber: 0.6g; Sugar: 5.1g; Fat 86% Protein 5% Carbs 9%

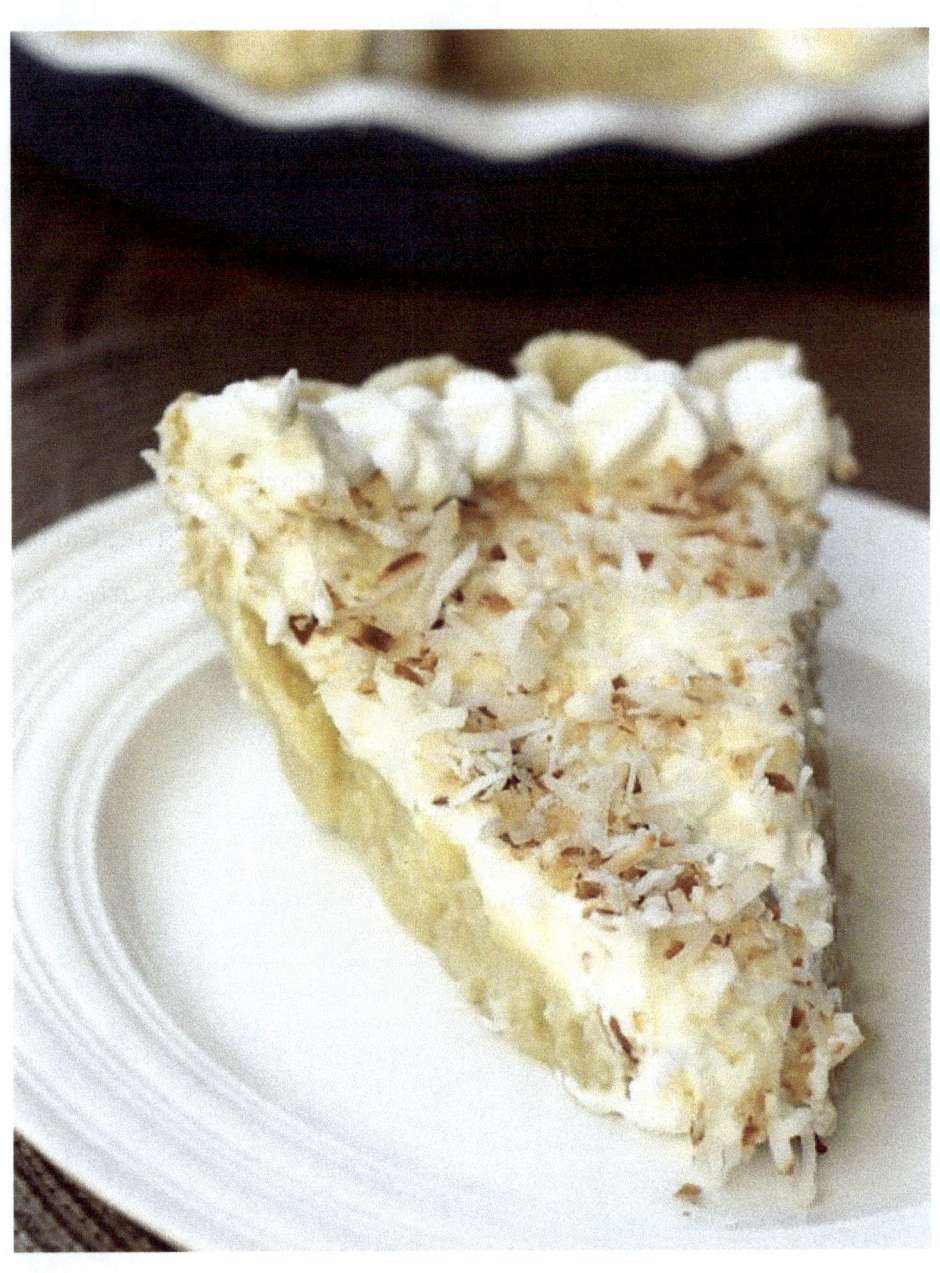

Delicious Pumpkin Cream Pie

Servings: 10

Cooking Time: 60 Minutes

Ingredients:

- For crust:
- 1 tsp erythritol
- 8 tbsp butter
- 1 ¼ cup almond flour
- Pinch of salt
- For filling:
- 2 eggs
- ½ tsp liquid stevia
- ½ cup erythritol
- 2 tbsp pumpkin pie spice
- ¼ cup sour cream
- ¾ cup heavy cream
- 15 oz can pumpkin puree

Directions:

1. For the crust: Preheat the oven to 350 F 0 C.
2. Add all crust ingredients into the food processor and process until dough is formed.
3. Transfer the dough in a pie dish and spread evenly.
4. Prick bottom on crust using fork or knife.
5. Bake crust in preheated oven for 10 minutes.

6. For the filling: Preheat the oven to 375 F 190 C.
7. In a large bowl, whisk eggs with sour cream, heavy cream, and pumpkin puree.
8. Add stevia, erythritol, and pumpkin pie spice and whisk well.
9. Pour cream pumpkin mixture into the baked crust and spread evenly.
10. Bake in preheated oven for 45-50 minutes.
11. Allow to cool completely then place in the refrigerator for 2-3 hours.
12. Serve and enjoy.

Nutrition Info: Per Servings: Net Carbs: 5.6g; Calories: 239; Total Fat: 21.8g; Saturated Fat: 9.5g Protein: 5.3g; Carbs: 8.3g; Fiber: 2.7g; Sugar: 2.1g; Fat 83% Protein 8% Carbs 9%

Flavorful Strawberry Cream Pie

Servings: 10

Cooking Time: 10 Minutes

Ingredients:

- 1 cup almond flour
- ¼ cup butter, melted
- 8 oz cream cheese, softened
- ½ cup erythritol
- ½ cup fresh strawberries
- ¾ cup heavy whipping cream

Directions:

1. In a bowl, mix together almond flour and melted butter.
2. Spread almond flour mixture into the pie dish evenly.
3. Add strawberries in a blender and blend until a smooth puree is formed.
4. Add strawberry puree in a large bowl.
5. Add remaining ingredients in a bowl and whisk until thick.
6. Transfer Strawberry cream mixture onto the pie crust and spread evenly.
7. Place in refrigerator for 2 hours.
8. Slice and serve.

Nutrition Info: Per Servings: Net Carbs: 2.5g; Calories: 217; Total Fat: 21.5g; Saturated Fat: 10.4g Protein: 4.4g; Carbs: 3.8g; Fiber: 1.3g; Sugar: 0.8g; Fat 88% Protein 8% Carbs 4%

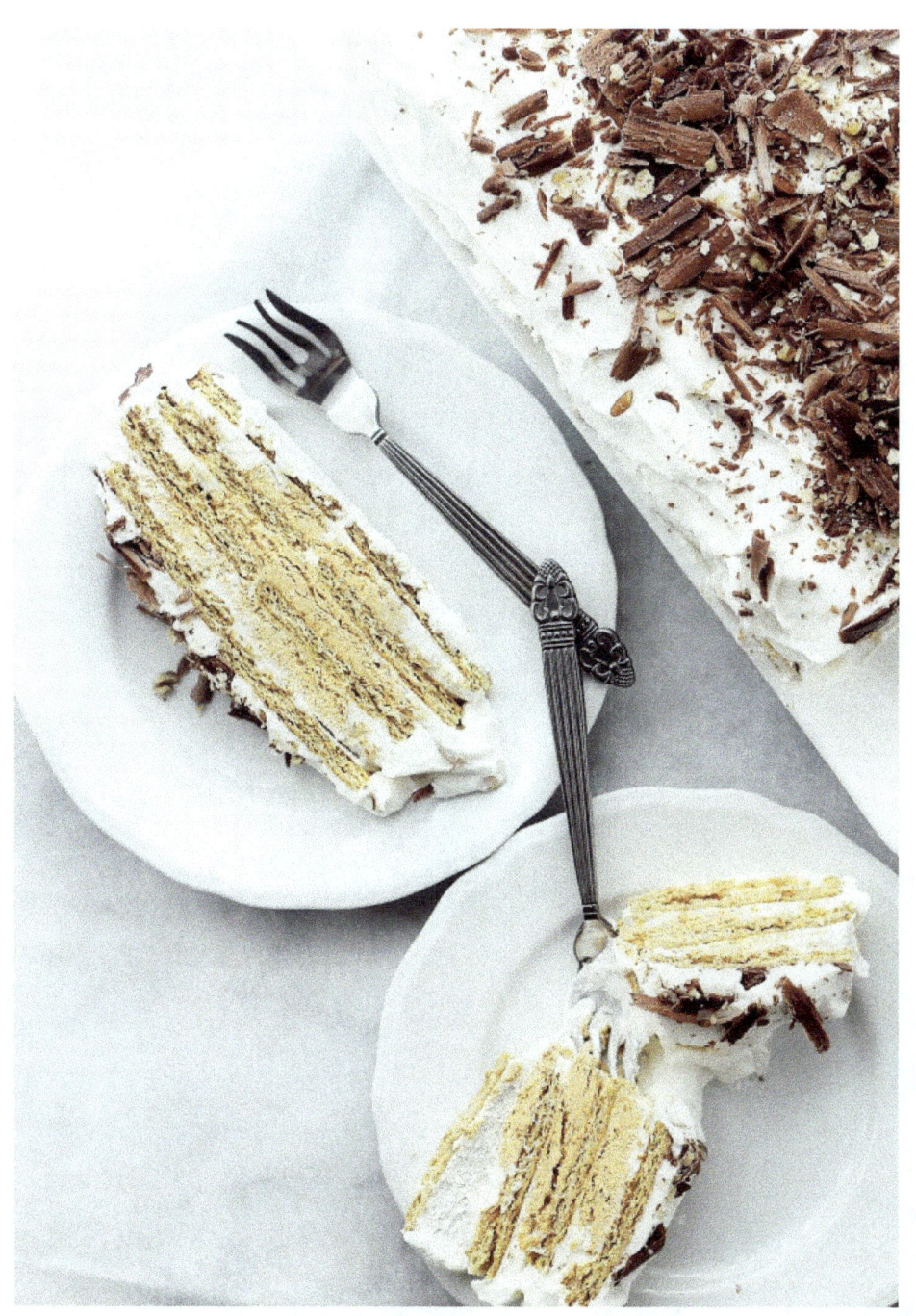

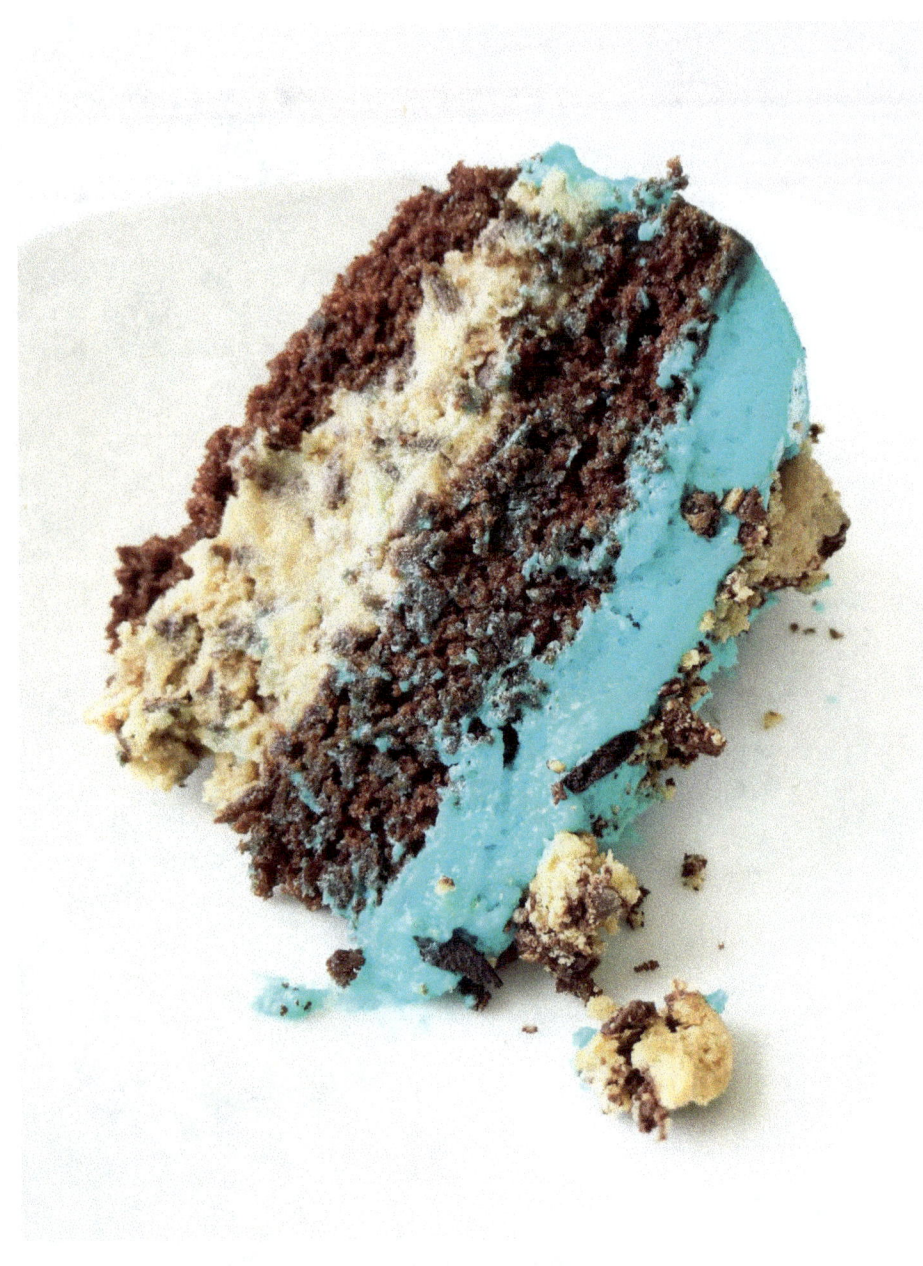

www.ingramcontent.com/pod-product-compliance
Lightning Source LLC
Chambersburg PA
CBHW071108030426
42336CB00013BA/1999